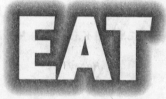

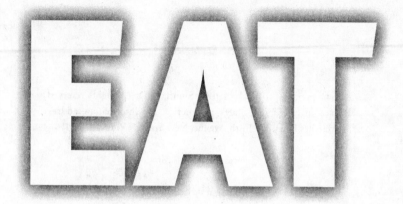

EAT

Feed Your Body and
Starve the Fat

IAN K. SMITH, M.D.

ST. MARTIN'S GRIFFIN
NEW YORK

www.stmartins.com

Design by Level C

Acknowledgments are given for some of the illustrative material used. The illustrations on pages 48 and 58, courtesy Oldways and the Whole Grains Council, wholegrainscouncil.org. The chart on page 153, first published in the *American Journal of Clinical Nutrition*, March 1, 2006, vol. 83, no. 529–542. Used with permission of the author, Barry Popkin.

Photographs are courtesy of the author unless otherwise noted.

The Library of Congress has cataloged the hardcover edition as follows:

Smith, Ian, 1969–
    Eat : the effortless weight loss solution / Ian K. Smith.—1st ed.
       p. cm.
    ISBN 978-0-312-54843-8 (hardback)
    1. Weight loss. I. Title.
    RM222.2.S6218 2011
    613.2'5—dc22

2010054464

ISBN 978-1-250-00428-4 (trade paperback)

First St. Martin's Griffin Edition: January 2012

10 9 8 7 6 5 4 3 2 1

To Robert Cherry, Jr. (Uncle Bob). You stood up when others sat down. You believed when others doubted. You opened your arms when others knotted them behind their backs. A *real* soldier. For that I will forever remain in your debt and love you from the deepest places that make my heart flutter.

And to my little team that wins the game of life for me every day: Tristé, Dashiell, and Declan. You give me purpose, hope, and more unconditional love than any human being deserves. Thank you so much for giving my life meaning.

Note to the Reader

This book is for informational purposes only. The author has endeavored to make sure it contains reliable and accurate information. However, research on diet and nutrition is evolving and subject to interpretation, and the conclusions presented here may differ from those found in other sources. As each individual's experience may vary, readers, especially those with existing health problems, should consult their physician or health care professional before adopting any nutritional changes based on information contained in this book. Individual readers are solely responsible for their own healthcare decisions, and the author and the publisher do not accept responsibility for any adverse effects individuals may claim to experience, whether directly or indirectly, based on information contained herein.

Contents

Acknowledgments

The work of an author is never a single-handed experience or effort. There are always names and faces of people the reading audience will never know, but who nonetheless have played a critical role in bringing my thoughts and words to the page. I honor those who have helped create and who have joined my 50 Million Pound Challenge and shared their inspiring journeys of weight loss. My personal assistants, Liza Rodriguez and Kathleen Biondi—thanks so much for making my life comfortable and keeping the train on track. I love you both. To my phenomenal family at St. Martin's Press—Elizabeth Beier (my eternally supportive and sharp-minded editor, who I selfishly never want to share with other authors), Michelle Richter (an editorial assistant whose skills and support I'm lucky to have benefited from on her way up), Steve Cohen (a horrific golfer, but awesome friend), Matthew Shear (a consistent believer), Sally Richardson (the Energizer Bunny), John Karle and John Murphy (titans of PR), Lorraine Saullo (the steady one who always says "yes"), Rob Grom (artist with a flair), and Edward Perez (the security guard in the lobby who thoughtfully grants me entrance with a nice smile and not a lot of typical New York City hassle). Lastly and most important, I must thank my biological family. None of this is possible without your inspiration and belief. Declan, Dashiell, Tristé, Storie (my darling niece), Jamie, Dana, Ma,

Acknowledgments

Pops, Uncle Johnny, Lynn, Aunt Bettie, Aunt Helen Gray, and Billy. I hope I continue to make good use of the love and skills that you all have instilled in me from my earliest days at Park Avenue Elementary School. Gramma—you gloriously continue to guide my heart.

*T*his is NOT a diet book.

If you're looking for a book that can improve the quality of your life, make you feel better, look better, lengthen your life—and YES, help you drop those stubborn excess pounds and maintain a healthy weight—then this is *the* book.

In *EAT,* you'll find scientifically based, easy-to-understand information about eating well and making smart decisions. The idea behind *EAT* is simple. Rather than instructing you to follow a rigid diet program that dictates every morsel you put into your mouth, I want to educate you on how to make your own decisions so that you feel free and empowered and *confident* when it comes to making food and lifestyle choices.

I decided to write this book for one simple reason: millions of people anxiously want to understand how to eat better—yet the advice that many experts dole out is either complicated or contradictory. I wanted to take the best research on healthful eating and boil it down so that after all of the fancy language and complex ideas have evaporated, what's left are the essentials of what it takes to eat better and feel better. Anyway, who really has the time or desire to read a 500-page encyclopedia on good eating?

This is not a diet book in the traditional sense. Instead, consider this a manual or crib notes on eating that will deliver all kinds of benefits. Yes, you will lose weight if you need to, but more than that, you can lower your blood pressure, reduce your cholesterol levels, increase your energy, feel younger, and fight all kinds of diseases simply by putting the right foods on your plate. Food is our body's fuel, and the purpose of this book is to teach you how to choose and mix this fuel to make sure you are filling up your body's tank with the highest octane available.

I've included charts that make it ridiculously easy for you to make smart food choices. Charts such as the Seafood Protein Sources or the Top 10 Antioxidant Fruits mean that all you have to do is pick from the list—you don't have to comb through a bunch of research papers and articles to create your own. At the end of each chapter is an **EAT Plan** with only a few simple suggestions you should follow to incorporate the message of that chapter into your life. I wanted you to have an actual plan to follow with instructions that are specific enough so that you don't feel as if there's a lot of work on your part to follow through with your good intentions in buying this book. I've purposely made the plan flexible enough that you can customize it according to your preferences.

Healthy eating will make you happier and can add years to your life. This does not mean, however, that you need to break the bank in order to provide your body with the best nourishment. The belief that "only the rich can eat well" is wrong on so many levels, and I hope this book will succeed in showing you why. "Food experts" tend to make the concept of healthy eating complicated. It's not. You don't need an advanced degree or personal chef—or even a lot of time—in order to put delicious and healthy food on the table.

What you need is simple. First, you need to want to eat well and enjoy the food you eat. Second, you need a basic understanding of food fundamentals that will quickly allow you to make decisions on your own—without having to consult a book, a nutritionist, or anyone else. Third, you need to *believe* that good eating is available to anyone who desires it, and not something accessible only to members of an exclusive club. *EAT* will give you the information and confidence you need to make eating fun, affordable, and life-enhancing.

Bon Appétit,

Ian K. Smith, M.D.

Follow the Rainbow 1

- ✦ Getting the Most Nutritional Bang for Your Buck
- ✦ The Power List: Fruits and Veggies You Must Have
- ✦ Colors Pack a Powerful Punch
- ✦ Antioxidants to the Rescue
- ✦ Fruits United for Weight Loss

*N*ature has made it easy for us to remember which foods provide the greatest nutritional punch. Think of the colors of the rainbow. It's that simple. Colorful foods are literally packed with all kinds of vitamins, minerals, and other nutrients that provide us with nutritional reinforcements to not only maintain the body's healthy status, but to fight off diseases that threaten our health. Fruits and vegetables are our greatest sources of health-promoting nutrients; however, we Americans largely ignore these critical natural health resources. A report by the Centers for Disease Control and Prevention (CDC) has shown that only 32.6 percent of American adults eat fruit two or more times a day. When it comes to vegetables, things are even worse. Only 27.2 percent of adults eat vegetables three or more times per day.[1]

Beyond vitamins and minerals, colorful fruits and vegetables are full of phytochemicals and antioxidants, two groups of disease-fighting, health-promoting compounds. Phytochemicals are natural compounds in plant food that work with nutrients and dietary fiber to protect against disease. Antioxidants are food compounds that neutralize or inactivate free radicals. These free radicals attack the body's cells and contribute to a variety of conditions including cancer, heart disease, and aging. Thankfully, there are lots of great-tasting fruits and vegetables that contain antioxidants and help reduce our risk for certain diseases. Loading up on antioxidant-rich foods is extremely important.

The benefits of a plant-based diet are abundantly available and clear. Several researchers have studied the eating and lifestyle habits of numerous populations around the world. They looked particularly carefully at the eating behaviors of those who lived the longest and had the best health. They found one critical component all of them shared: their diets were high in fruits, vegetables, and legumes and low in red meat. The CDC buttressed this research with a report that showed Americans who ate a more plant-based diet also had the lowest Body Mass Index (BMI), which meant a reduced risk of the many health problems associated with being overweight.

Let's be clear. Eating a health*ier* diet does not mean you have to go to the other extreme and become a vegetarian. There is a very comfortable middle ground that can be achieved by eating more fruits and vegetables and also choosing more poultry and fish, and making red meat an occasional meal. To better understand how to choose the best fruits and vegetables to give you the advantage you're looking for, you need to understand just a few basics.

Nutrient Density

You don't have to become a medical doctor or registered dietician—or even visit one—to know how to make smart food choices. The relatively new concept of "nutrient density," or "nutrient richness," is easy to understand and can immediately improve the quality of your life. Nutrient density refers to the amount of nutrients contained within a given volume of food. Foods that are high in nutrients and low in calories are considered "nutrient dense." Foods that have few nutrients and are high in calories are considered to be "nutrient poor." By simply making sure that 75 percent of what you eat is nutrient dense, you will see dramatic physical changes as well as an almost immediate energy boost.

You can also look specifically at the density of one nutrient. Let's say you feel a cold coming on and you're interested in boosting your intake of vitamin C. You would look for foods that are nutrient dense in vitamin C. Bell peppers have 174 milligrams of vitamin C per cup and only 25 calories. But fried onion rings contain less than 1 milligram of vitamin C per cup and have 200 calories. The recommended daily value intake of vitamin C is 60 milligrams. That means it would take only a third of a cup of bell peppers to meet that requirement and only a little more than 8 calories to go along with it. However, it would take more than 15,000 calories of fried onion rings to meet the recommended 60 milligrams of vitamin C. The bell peppers are nutrient dense and the onion rings are nutrient poor.

You're between meals and your stomach is growling for a snack. You have a choice: go to the vending machine and get a shiny red apple, or pluck a glazed doughnut from a box that someone has conveniently brought to your office and left out for everyone. It's common knowledge that the apple is the healthier choice, but why? Apples are chock-full of vitamins, fiber, and phytonutrients that will keep you healthy. Doughnuts have almost no nutritional value whatsoever. An apple answers a craving not just with lots of healthy nutrients, but on only 80 calories. The doughnut, however, is not only bare of nutrients, but it will also load 200 calories into your system. The apple is nutrient dense and the doughnut is nutrient poor.

To make it easy for you to make the best food choices, here's a list of the most nutrient-dense fruits and vegetables.

Nutrient-Dense Fruits

Apples	Oranges
Apricots	Papaya
Avocados	Pears
Bananas	Pineapple
Blueberries	Plums
Cranberries	Prunes
Figs	Raisins
Grapefruit	Raspberries
Grapes	Strawberries
Kiwi	Tomatoes
Lemons	Watermelon

Nutrient-Dense Vegetables

Asparagus	Leeks
Bell peppers	Mustard greens
Broccoli	Onions
Cabbage	Spinach
Carrots	Squash
Celery	Sweet potatoes
Eggplant	Turnip greens
Green beans	

Your Daily Fruit Consumption Recommendation

For many years, the U.S. Department of Agriculture (USDA) has made recommendations concerning the major categories of food products and how much of them we should consume to maintain a healthy diet. The USDA food pyramid, established in 1992 but based on repeatedly modified versions of the 1917 food guide, has been the official guide to achieving this objective. Most people know this pyramid exists, but few really know what it says and even fewer actually follow its recommendations. In 2010, the USDA modified the pyramid so that it's easier to understand and more relevant to today's way of living. Below is the new recommendation for daily fruit intake.

Daily Fruit Intake Recommendation

Children	2–3 years old	1 cup
	4–8 years old	1–1.5 cups
Girls	9–13 years old	1.5 cups
	14–18 years old	1.5 cups
Boys	9–13 years old	1.5 cups
	14–18 years old	2 cups
Women	19–30 years old	2 cups
	31–50 years old	1.5 cups
	51+ years old	1.5 cups
Men	19–30 years old	2 cups
	31–50 years old	2 cups
	51+ years old	2 cups

Source: USDA, www.mypyramid.gov

These amounts are appropriate for individuals who get less than 30 minutes per day of moderate physical activity, beyond normal daily activities. Those who are more physically active may be able to consume more while staying within calorie needs.

The USDA offers even more guidance in reaching your fruit consumption goals: 1 cup from the fruit group can be 1 cup of fruit, 1 cup of 100 percent fruit juice, or ½ cup of dried fruit. Below are a few examples of what would constitute a cup of fruit.

	Amount That Counts as 1 Cup of Fruit
Apple	½ large (3.25" diameter) 1 small (2.5" diameter) 1 cup sliced or chopped, raw or cooked
Applesauce	1 cup
Banana	1 large
Cantaloupe	1 cup diced or melon balls
Dried fruit (raisins, prunes, etc.)	½ cup dried fruit
100% fruit juice (orange, apple, grape, grapefruit, etc.)	1 cup
Grapefruit	1 medium (4" diameter) 1 cup sections

	Amount That Counts as 1 Cup of Fruit
Grapes	1 cup whole or cut up (32 seedless)
Orange	1 large (3$\frac{1}{16}$" diameter) or 1 cup sections
Peach	1 large (2$\frac{3}{4}$" diameter) 1 cup sliced or diced, raw, cooked, or canned, drained 2 halves canned
Pear	1 medium 1 cup sliced or diced, raw, cooked, or canned, drained
Pineapple	1 cup chunks, sliced or crushed, raw, cooked or canned, drained
Plum	1 cup sliced, raw or cooked 3 medium or 2 large plums
Strawberries	8 large

Your Daily Vegetable Consumption Recommendation

It's not an earth-shattering revelation that we should eat vegetables every day. But even with years of national headlines and health campaigns to encourage Americans to eat more veggies, we have been falling down on the job. In fact, according to a recent report from the CDC, only 26 percent of adults eat vegetables three or more times a day. This is less than we were eating ten years ago. The health benefits of a plant-based diet have been well documented, yet Americans still turn to meat and fried foods first. According to the USDA, Americans eat more than 220 pounds of meat per year per person, an astounding doubling of the global average. And our carnivorous habits have gotten worse: meat consumption has increased more than 50 percent since 1950.

So how many vegetables should we eat? The USDA has modified its recommendations and created a simple chart to follow.

Daily Vegetable Intake Recommendation

Children	2–3 years old	1 cup
	4–8 years old	1.5 cups
Girls	9–13 years old	2 cups
	14–18 years old	2.5 cups
Boys	9–13 years old	2.5 cups
	14–18 years old	3 cups
Women	19–30 years old	2.5 cups
	31–50 years old	2.5 cups
	51+ years old	2 cups

Daily Vegetable Intake Recommendation		
Men	19–30 years old	3 cups
	31–50 years old	3 cups
	51+ years old	2.5 cups

Source: USDA, www.mypyramid.gov

These amounts are appropriate for individuals who get less than 30 minutes per day of moderate physical activity, beyond normal daily activities. Those who are more physically active may be able to consume more while staying within calorie needs.

So what counts as a cup of vegetables? According to the USDA, 1 cup of raw or cooked vegetables, 1 cup of vegetable juice, or 2 cups of raw leafy greens can be considered as 1 cup from the vegetable group. Here are some other examples of what serves as a cup of vegetables.

	Amount That Counts as 1 Cup of Vegetables
Bean sprouts	1 cup cooked
Broccoli	1 cup chopped or florets 3 spears 5" long, raw or cooked
Cabbage, green	1 cup, chopped or shredded, raw or cooked
Carrots	1 cup strips, slices, or chopped 2 medium carrots 1 cup baby carrots (about 12)
Cauliflower	1 cup pieces of florets, raw or cooked

continued

	Amount That Counts as 1 Cup of Vegetables
Celery	1 cup, diced or sliced, raw or cooked 2 large stalks (11" to 17" long)
Corn, yellow or white	1 cup 1 large ear (8–9 inches)
Cucumbers	1 cup raw, sliced or chopped
Dry beans and peas (black, garbanzo, kidney, pinto, soy, split peas, black-eyed peas)	1 cup whole or mashed, cooked
Green or red peppers	1 cup chopped, raw or cooked 1 large pepper (3" diameter, $3\frac{3}{4}$" long)
Green or wax beans	1 cup cooked
Green peas	1 cup
Greens (collards, mustard greens, turnip greens, kale)	1 cup cooked
Lettuce, iceberg or head	2 cups raw, shredded, or chopped
Mushrooms	1 cup raw or cooked

	Amount That Counts as 1 Cup of Vegetables
Onions	1 cup chopped, raw or cooked
Raw leafy greens: spinach, romaine, watercress, dark green leafy lettuce	2 cups raw
Spinach	1 cup cooked 2 cups raw
Summer squash or Zucchini	1 cup cooked, sliced or diced
Sweet potato	1 large baked ($2\frac{1}{4}$" or more diameter) 1 cup sliced or mashed, cooked
Tomatoes	1 large raw whole (3") 1 cup chopped or sliced, raw, canned, or cooked
Winter squash (acorn, butternut, hubbard)	1 cup cubed, cooked

The Rainbow Breakdown of Foods

When it comes to choosing the healthiest foods, don't clutter your mind with all of the technical nutritional jargon and scientific analyses. Leave that to the experts. Sometimes just keeping it simple can do the trick. Whether you're ordering food at a restaurant or sitting down to eat at home, remember this: "Eat a rainbow and find a pot of health gold." Go for the color and you can't go wrong. Below you'll find what each color group will give you and some examples that you should try.

Reds

There are plenty of red fruits and vegetables that are easily accessible, tasty, inexpensive, and pack a powerful nutritional punch. Consuming these foods in abundance will only give you a kick in the right direction when it comes to loading up on vitamins, minerals, and other nutrients. The red coloring is due to natural pigments called "anthocyanins" and "lycopene." Anthocyanins are typically found in strawberries, red raspberries, red grapes, red onions, and other red fruits and vegetables. They are strong antioxidants that protect our body's cells from damage. Lycopene can be found in such foods as tomatoes, pink grapefruit, and watermelon. It's best absorbed by the body when the food is cooked, such as the tomatoes in spaghetti sauce. Lycopene is believed to reduce the risk of several types of cancer, particularly prostate cancer. Choose from some examples of the red group below.

The Reds

Beets	Red apples
Cherries	Red bell peppers
Cranberries	Red cabbage
Guava	Red grapes
Papaya	Rhubarb
Pink grapefruit	Strawberries
Pomegranates	Tomatoes
Radishes	Watermelon
Raspberries	

Oranges/Yellows

These fruits and vegetables owe their alluring color to the natural plant pigments called "carotenoids." The most common carotenoids in the North American diet are alpha-carotene, beta-carotene, beta-cryptoxanthin, lutein, zeaxanthin, and lycopene. Beta-carotene gets the most attention and rightfully so. It is found in a variety of foods, including carrots, sweet potatoes, and pumpkins. The body converts beta-carotene into vitamin A, which helps form and maintain healthy teeth, skeletal and soft tissue, mucous membranes, and skin. It's most famous for promoting good vision, which is why our parents always said, "Eat your carrots for healthy eyes." The active form of vitamin A is called retinol and it produces the pigments in the retina of the eye.

Carotenoids are believed to be good for your heart: studies have shown that people who consume a diet high in these foods had a much lower risk of heart attack and death compared to those who ate few carotenoid-containing foods. One study even showed that those who ate a diet high in carotenoid-rich vegetables were 43 percent less likely to develop age-related macular degeneration, a disorder that can lead to blindness. Below are some examples of the orange/yellow group.

Orange/Yellow Group

Apricots	Pineapple
Cantaloupe	Plantains
Carrots	Squash
Corn	Sweet potatoes
Kumquats	Tangerines
Lemons	Yellow pears
Mango	Yellow peppers
Oranges	Yellow tomatoes
Peaches	Yellow watermelon

Greens

Remember those elementary school science classes where you learned about chlorophyll and its important role in photosynthesis, where plants emit the critical oxygen we breathe? Well, it's that same chlorophyll that gives green fruits and vegetables their color. Some members of the green group, such as spinach and other dark leafy greens, celery, cucumbers, green peppers, and peas, contain an important compound called lutein. It's believed that lutein helps prevent eye diseases including age-related macular degeneration, cataracts, and retinitis pigmentosa. While more studies need to be conducted to confirm its other benefits, many scientists believe it can help prevent colon cancer, breast cancer, type 2 diabetes, and heart disease. Below is a list of some examples from this group.

Green Group

Artichoke	Green onions
Asparagus	Honeydew melon
Bok choy	Kale
Broccoli	Kiwi
Brussels sprouts	Lime
Cabbage	Okra
Celery	Romaine lettuce
Collard greens	Spinach
Cucumbers	Turnip greens
Green bell pepper	Zucchini

Members of this group also contain a group of antioxidants called indoles, which are believed to help protect against some types of cancer. Indoles can be found in broccoli, cauliflower, cabbage, brussels sprouts, bok choy, arugula, turnips, rutabaga, and other cruciferous vegetables.

Leafy green vegetables in this group are also rich in a B vitamin called folate, a compound important for pregnant women to consume to prevent birth defects in the newborn, which are called neural tube defects and affect the brain and spinal cord. The two most common defects are spina bifida and anencephaly (much of brain doesn't develop).

Blues/Purples

The fruits and vegetables in this group are colored by the natural plant pigments anthocyanins. Found in such foods as grapes, raisins, blueberries, and blackberries, these compounds function as powerful antioxidants that protect cells from damage. Some evidence suggests that they can be helpful in reducing the risk for some serious diseases, such as heart disease, cancer, and stroke. Below is a list of some of the foods in this group.

Blue/Purple Group

Blackberries	Prunes
Blueberries	Purple cabbage
Eggplant	Purple grapes
Figs	Raisins
Plums	

Frozen Fruits and Veggies

Many people—doctors, nutritionists, and "foodies"—would have you believe that frozen fruits and veggies are either unhealthy or not as nutritious as fresh ones. The truth, however, is that these frozen goodies can be equally healthy depending on the manufacturer and process used to freeze the goods. Make sure you read the package carefully to detect whether additives have been included in the freezing process. Be particularly on the lookout for sodium (salt). Most people don't know that manufacturers often add a significant amount of salt to foods, quantities so large sometimes that on their own they can cause you to exceed your daily sodium recommendation.

Frozen fruits and veggies are also useful when you need a quick snack, because they are fast foods that are good for you. I am not ashamed, after a long day, to reach into the freezer and pull out a bag of frozen veggies. My family happens to enjoy the Birds Eye Steamfresh Corn and Mixed Vegetables. Not only are they ready to eat in four minutes or less, but they are nutritious and very tasty. Frozen fruits are excellent because they travel well and keep over long periods of time. You can pack them as a snack, and if your destination doesn't have refrigeration available, it doesn't matter. Your fruit will be ready to eat as it is or ready to be added to all types of foods, including salads, cereal, and yogurt.

Best Antioxidants

Now that you understand the importance of antioxidants and the potential benefits they can bring us, how do you find out which fruits and vegetables pack the greatest antioxidant punch? Thanks to researchers at the Human Nutrition Research Center on Aging at Tufts University, finding out is simple. Here are the top ten antioxidant performers. Take your pick.

Top 10 Antioxidant Fruits

Prunes	Raspberries
Raisins	Plums
Blueberries	Oranges
Blackberries	Red grapes
Strawberries	Cherries

Top 10 Antioxidant Vegetables

Kale	Beets
Spinach	Red bell peppers
Brussels sprouts	Onions
Alfalfa sprouts	Corn
Broccoli flowers	Eggplant

Fiber

Fiber is extremely important in our diets and the majority of Americans simply don't get enough of it. The health benefits of fiber are numerous, including reducing the risk for diabetes and heart disease, as well as maintaining bowel integrity and health. The National Academy of Sciences' Institute of Medicine sets this recommendation for how much fiber we should consume on a daily basis.

	Age 50 and Younger	Age 51 and Older
Men	38 grams	30 grams
Women	25 grams	21 grams

Fiber is found mostly in whole grains, vegetables, legumes, and fruits. (For a more in-depth look at fiber, see chapter 4.) Some fruits are particularly high in fiber content. The top ten are listed below.

Fruit	Calories	Grams of Fiber per 100 Calories
Raspberries, 1 cup	60	8.0
Blackberries, 1 cup	74	7.6
Strawberries, 1 cup	45	3.4
Prunes, ½ cup, cooked	113	7.0

continued

Fruit	Calories	Grams of Fiber per 100 Calories
Papaya, 1 medium	118	5.5
Orange, 1 medium	50	3.0
Apple, 1 medium	81	3.7
Pears, 1 medium	98	4.0
Figs, dried, 5	237	8.5
Avocado, half	150	4.0

Fruits to Lose Weight

You've probably heard of the glycemic index (GI) scale. Nutritionists and diet experts have embraced this classification of foods because it can be a powerful guide to not only making smarter food choices, but also to help you lose weight. I don't want to bore you with the enormous amount of scientific details that explain how the index works, so I'll cut to the chase. The glycemic index is a way of ranking foods based on how fast the body breaks them down into simple sugar, which you might also know as glucose. The faster a food is broken down into sugar, the faster and higher the levels of sugar rise in the blood. The faster your blood sugar levels rise, the stronger the signal to your pancreas to release the hormone known as insulin. The release of too much insulin at once or several times throughout the day can lead to weight gain because it increases your body's absorption of sugar, and if this sugar isn't used right away, it's converted to fat. So beyond just considering the calories within food, it's also helpful to consider the glycemic index. The lower the glycemic index, the better the food when it comes to weight loss.

Best Weight-Loss Fruits per Glycemic Index

Fruit	GI
Cherries (raw sour)	22
Grapefruit	25
Apricots (dried)	30
Apples	38
Pears	38
Plums	39
Peaches	42
Kiwi	47
Oranges	48
Grapes	49

Note: A high GI = 70 and above, medium GI = 56–69, low GI = 55 and under

Vitamin C

This popular vitamin also goes by the name ascorbic acid. It's a water-soluble vitamin that is critical for our bodies to function normally. Whether it's forming collagen tissue; building healthy bones, teeth, and blood vessels; or absorbing iron and calcium, vitamin C plays a role. Humans can't produce vitamin C, so it's essential that we get it from what we eat and drink. The daily recommended intake is 90 milligrams per day for adult men and 75 milligrams per day for adult women.[2] The common perception is that oranges are the best source of vitamin C. When you have a cold, someone has probably suggested drinking orange juice to load up on vitamin C. To most people's surprise, however, oranges aren't even in the top three of vitamin C–containing fruits. Take a look at the list on page 25.

Food	Serving Size	Amount of Vit. C (mg)
Papaya	1	187.9
Bell peppers	1 cup	174.8
Broccoli	1 cup	123.4
Brussels sprouts	1 cup	96.7
Strawberries	1 cup	81.7
Oranges	1	69.7
Cantaloupe	1 cup	67.5
Grapefruit	½	66.0
Kiwi	1	57.0

Top 10 Fruits Overall

There are many ways to measure and assess the nutritional quality of fruits. Ask fifty different nutritionists and they'll give you fifty different lists of what they consider to be the healthiest fruits. After scouring numerous lists, I found that there were several fruits that appeared on most of them. The list I found to be most thorough and best backed-up was published by the Center for Science in the Public Interest. They ranked fruits based on six nutrients plus carotenoids. The fruits listed on the next page are considered to be gold medalists.

There are some health advocates who suggest you consume nine servings of fruit and vegetables each day. By all accounts, this is a rather ambitious goal and one most people are unlikely to reach. If you can get that much in, great, but if you can't, you haven't failed. Eating five servings of fruits and vegetables each day is an effective way to balance your diet and reap the health benefits that these super foods offer.

Top 10 Fruits

Guava	Cantaloupe
Watermelon	Orange
Grapefruit, pink or red	Strawberries
Kiwifruit	Apricots
Papaya	Blackberries

Source: *Nutrition Action Health Letter,* May 1998,
from Center for Science In the Public Interest.

Tips for Adding Fruits and Veggies to Your Diet

✦ Each weekend take cut-up fresh or frozen fruits. Make mini-fruit salads by placing mixed fruits either in a baggie or plastic cup with a lid. Make enough so that you will have at least one for each day.

✦ Peppers, baby carrots, sliced cucumbers, and celery travel extremely well. Fill a snack bag with a mixture of them and use each bag as a snack when those hunger pangs hit.

✦ Make your own smoothies or buy them to order. Make sure you don't add many extra ingredients that will increase the calories. Try adding things like ice chips, low-fat yogurt, bananas, or a cup of orange juice.

EAT Plan

✦ Eat 5 servings of fruits and vegetables each day. Choose them from the nutrient-dense lists in this chapter (page 8). Variety is helpful. Every day choose two different fruits from your list so that consecutive days don't have the same fruit.

✦ Every other day try to consume 1 cup (8 ounces) of freshly squeezed fruit juice or vegetable juice. One day it might be tomato, another day orange, and the next beet juice. Mix it up so that you don't get bored.

✦ Try to vary the fruits and vegetables you consume from one day to the next. Choose strategically. Every day at least one of your servings should come from the list of high-fiber foods (pages 21–22) and one should come from the lists of antioxidant fruits and vegetables (pages 20–21).

✦ If possible, always eat the skin of your fruit. The skin contains a disproportionate amount of the fruit's nutrients. But make sure you wash the skin before eating it.

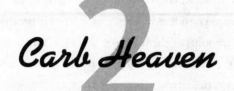

Carb Heaven

- ✦ Carbs: The Good vs. the Evil
- ✦ Carb-Counting Conundrum
- ✦ Beating the Sugar Monster
- ✦ Become a World-Class Food Detective

*O*ne of the greatest crimes ever perpetrated against the public interest and a food particle has been committed over the last decade. The innocent victim is a class of macronutrients called carbohydrates—carbs in today's vernacular. This extremely valuable resource has taken an undeserved beating from fly-by-night fad diets and purveyors of misinformation who have tried to convince the world that carbs are the number one food enemy, responsible for the outrageous levels of obesity in the industrialized world.

The truth is that carbs are critical to life and without them we simply would not survive. Carbs are one of the three macronutrients—along

with fat and protein—in our diets. They are called macronutrients because we need them in large (*macro*) supply in order to live. (Vitamins
and minerals are considered to be micronutrients because we require
small [*micro*] amounts of them for our bodies to function properly.) As
important as macronutrients are, carbs are the most important because
we need them in the largest amounts.

Carbohydrates are the fuel of life. They are the body's primary
source of energy. All of the tissues and cells in our body can use
glucose—the basic unit of a carbohydrate—for energy. The brain,
central nervous system, kidneys, and muscles are particularly depen-
dent on carbohydrates to function properly. Muscles and the liver
store carbohydrates so they can be used later when the body needs
energy. You might've heard of this stored form: it's called glycogen.
When the body's energy needs increase, let's say while running a
marathon, then glycogen is released from storage—in the liver and/
or muscles—into the blood, where it is then subsequently broken down
to be used as energy.

Carbohydrates also provide nutrients for the friendly bacteria that
live in our intestinal tract, where they maintain our intestinal health as
well as assist in proper waste elimination. What many people don't know
is that carbs are also important in helping the body absorb calcium, an
important mineral that keeps our bones and teeth healthy as well as our
heart beating rhythmically and the blood, nerves, and muscles functioning correctly. It's unfortunate and potentially harmful that carbs
have gotten such a bad rap in recent years. Carbs are by no means perfect, and like most other things, some are good and some are bad, but
unlike the proverbial rotten apples in the barrel, bad carbs shouldn't be
allowed to spoil the good carbs.

What Exactly Is a Carbohydrate?

Many people throw around the words "carb" and "carbohydrate" but don't have a good understanding of what they mean. The basics first. Carbohydrates are everywhere and in almost every food, so it's extremely difficult to go the entire day without eating some. Carbohydrates are compounds comprised of carbon, hydrogen, and oxygen that are a food source of energy for plants, animals, and humans. You might've forgotten your fourth-grade earth science, but carbohydrates originate either directly or indirectly from plants through a process called photosynthesis, where the sun's light energy is used by the chlorophyll (the substance that makes leaves green) to synthesize water (from the soil) and carbon dioxide (from the air) into glucose, or sugar.

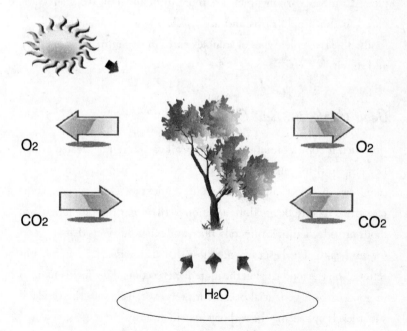

O_2 O_2

CO_2 CO_2

H_2O

The *only* carbohydrates that don't come from plants are those found in dairy products, such as the sugar found in milk: lactose.

There are two major forms of carbohydrates—simple and complex—and they are classified based on their chemical structure and how quickly the sugar is digested and absorbed. Simple carbohydrates are also called simple sugars. They have one (single) or two (double) sugars that are easy to digest and have little nutritional value. They include such sugars as fructose (found in fruits), glucose (found in corn, rice, potatoes, etc.), lactose (found in dairy), sucrose (table sugar), and galactose (found in milk products). Simple carbs are also found in whole fruits.

Complex carbohydrates are also called starches. They are comprised of three or more sugars that are typically strung together in long chains that can be hundreds or thousands of units long, thus the label "complex." Complex carbohydrates are more difficult to digest when compared to the simple carbs and are *typically* associated with healthier foods. The two chief types of complex carbs in the human diet are fiber and starch.

Good Carbs vs. Bad Carbs

When it comes to nutritional value, all carbs are not created equal. For ease of distinguishing these carbs we have divided them into the categories of "good" and "bad" (see list on next page). In general, complex carbs tend to be good. In addition to the sugar they contain, these foods provide vitamins, minerals, fiber, and other nutrients that are good for our health. The best carbs are those that are *unrefined*. Look for "unrefined" on the food label in the ingredients section. The fiber contained in good carbs is beneficial because it prevents the sudden rise of blood sugar levels by causing the carbohydrate to be absorbed more slowly.

Good Carbs	Bad Carbs
Fruits	Soda
Whole-grain cereals	Cookies
Brown rice	Cake
Whole-grain breads	Fruit drinks (not 100% juice)
Low-fat dairy	Frozen desserts
Vegetables	White rice
Beans	White pasta
Legumes	Jelly
Raw nuts	Most puddings
Seeds	Alcohol
Whole-grain pasta	Pastries/Danishes
Juice, freshly squeezed with no additives	

In most cases, simple carbohydrates tend to make up the group we consider to be bad carbs. These foods typically include *processed* and *refined* sugars that can be found in candy, carbonated beverages, syrups, and table sugar. Refined sugars are made from raw sugarcane or raw sugar beets. Through a lengthy purification process of washing, boiling, centrifuging, filtering, and drying, the vast majority of the nutritional elements contained in the sugar plant are stripped away along with impurities from the raw sugar, leaving sucrose, the white granulated sweetener you know as table sugar. This is why simple carbohydrate foods tend to be highly caloric, but have virtually no nutritional value—it's all been stripped away.

While most simple carbohydrates are bad because they come stripped of healthy nutrients, those found in fruits, dairy, and vegetables are an exception to the rule. Some of these food products contain simple carbs, but these are also accompanied by other healthy nutrients such as vitamins, minerals, and phytonutrients.

How Many Carbs Do You Need?

To understand how ridiculously misguided all the hype about carbs being the enemy and the benefits of no-carb or low-carb diets has been, all you have to do is look at the current recommendation for daily carbohydrate intake. According to the Institute of Medicine of the National Academies, based on a 2,000-calorie-per-day diet, 45 to 60 percent of an adult's daily calories should come from carbohydrates—while 20 to 35 percent should come from fat and 10 to 35 percent should come from protein.

They also recommend that the bulk of these carbohydrates be complex carbs rather than simple carbs and worthless refined sugar. It seems to be a popular sport to gang up on carbohydrates as the cause of the international spreading of waistlines, but the truth is that it's much more than carbs that has led to the obesity epidemic. At the top of the list is portion control. The caloric intake in a typical Western diet is so far out of control that most people don't know what appropriate serving sizes even look like (see chapter 7, "Size Matters").

Yes, there are carbs you'd do best to avoid, but to avoid *all* carbohydrates is a mistake that will eventually catch up with your body. Remember, the only way to get the healthy fiber our body needs is through carbohydrates—plant foods. Making them the only or biggest culprit for our weight problems is a diversion from the simple truth: we're eating too much, making bad food choices, and not exercising anywhere near as much as we should be to achieve and maintain a healthy weight. In fact, when you compare carbs to other macronutrients and popular alcohol, you learn the true story about where our calories are *really* coming from and why blaming carbs is convenient but not completely honest. Take note of fat and alcohol.

The True Calorie Counter	
Protein	4 calories per gram
Carbohydrates	4 calories per gram
Alcohol	7 calories per gram
Fat	9 calories per gram

Added Sugars: Your Enemy

If there is one thing that this anticarb movement has gotten right, it's the vilification of added sugars. These are the sugars and syrups that are added to foods and beverages during the manufacturing process or at the table. Added sugars are *not* the naturally occurring sugars found in milks and fruits. Sugars are added to products for one reason: to satisfy the common taste appeal we have for sweet foods and drinks. Added sugars are the worst of the worst and should be avoided as much as possible, or at most consumed in very modest quantities.

According to the American Heart Association (AHA), people who consume too much added sugar are at greater risk for obesity and high blood pressure, both of which in turn are strong risk factors for cardiovascular disease. Thus, the AHA has come out with guidelines for added sugar consumption. Their recommendation is that we consume no more than 100 calories per day from added sugar; this is equal to about 6 teaspoons of table sugar. Just as a point of reference, one can of regular soda has eight teaspoons of sugar in the form of high fructose corn syrup. This is why it's so critical to be able to read the food labels of what you're eating (more on this on page 36).

Foods/Beverages Containing the Most Added Sugars

- Candy
- Cookies
- Pies
- Cakes
- Regular soft drinks (sodas)
- Fruit drinks (such as fruit punch or juice blends)
- Grain products (such as sweet rolls and cinnamon toast)
- Milk-based desserts (such as ice cream, sweetened yogurt, and sweetened milk)

Source: USDA

Too Much Sugar

Despite our need to consume appropriate amounts of carbohydrates, one thing is for sure: Americans consume far too many added sugars, and it's gotten worse over the last decade. How bad is it? Imagine thirty-one 5-pound bags of sugar sitting on your kitchen table.

According to the USDA, that's how much each of us consumes on average each year. Twenty-nine of the 155 pounds that we consume come from our sugar bowls. The rest is hidden in different foods: candy, soda, junk foods, syrups, sauces, breads, or condiments like ketchup.

The numbers are staggering. According to the USDA, each day the average adult eats approximately 20 teaspoons of added sugar. This adds up to about 320 calories. For people trying to lose weight on a 1,500-calorie-per-day diet, that's as many as 20 percent of their calories in added sugars—wasted calories that won't fill them up. And to make matters even worse, these empty calories deliver virtually *no* nutritional value.

The major source of these added sugars is soda, delivering an astounding 33 percent of the added sugar we eat and drink. Twenty-six percent comes from a variety of prepared foods such as ketchup, peanut butter, and canned fruits and vegetables. Sweetened fruit drinks account for 10 percent of the total added sugars we consume, followed by cake and candy, which come in at 5 percent each, then ready-to-eat cereals at 4 percent.

Become a Smart Food Detective: Read the Label

We would instantly become better eaters if we simply put to use one of our most valuable life skills: reading. For whatever reason, whether we're too busy or we're intimidated by the scientific terms and columns of numbers, we simply don't spend enough time looking at food labels and getting a basic understanding of what the products we eat contain. The fine print on the back of the can or box isn't for anyone else—it's for *you*, the consumer. It's really not as difficult as you might think to get the information you need. It simply requires a couple of minutes of your time to flip the package over and pick out a couple of terms. Take a look at this food label from a can of barley soup.

Nutrition Facts
Serving Size: 1 cup (245g)
Servings Per Container: about 2

Amount Per Serving
Calories 130   Calories from Fat 15

	% Daily Value
Total Fat 1.5 g	2%
Saturated Fat 0g	0%
Trans Fat 0g	
Cholesterol 0mg	0%
Sodium 400 mg	17%
Total Carbohydrate 24g	8%
Dietary Fiber 5g	20%
Sugars 2g	
Protein 6g	

Vitamin A 6%	Vitamin C 0%
Calcium 6%	Iron 15%

*Percent Daily Values are based on a 2,000 calorie diet. Your daily values may be higher or lower depending on your calorie needs:

	Calories:	2,000	2,500
Total Fat	Less than	65g	80g
Saturated Fat	Less than	20g	25g
Cholesterol	Less than	300mg	300mg
Sodium	Less than	2,400mg	2,400mg
Total Carbohydate		300g	375g
Dietary Fiber		25g	30g

Calories per gram:
Fat 9   Carbohydrate 4   Protein 4

The very first thing you should pay attention to is how many servings are contained within the package you're holding. The sample above, says there are "2" servings in this can. That means if you ate the entire can of soup, you're not eating a single serving of soup, you're actually eating two servings.

Once you have established the number of servings contained in the package, remember that all of the ingredients listed and their values are for only *one* serving, not the entire package. I think you should always take a look at the calories first. So, the calorie count for one serving of this soup is 130. You might look at this and say, "Wow, that's not too bad. I can eat cans of this stuff and not pack in many calories." Slow down: those 130 calories are how many calories there are *per serving*. We've already discovered that the can of soup contains two servings. To figure out the calorie count for the entire can, all we need is our third-grade math:

Total calories = (number of servings) × (the number of calories
  per serving)
Total calories = 2 × 130
Total calories = 260 calories

Your total intake from that can of soup is 260 calories. While this number certainly isn't off-the-chart, it's substantial enough to consider and if you're counting calories, it's definitely much more than the 130 calories you might have thought when you first read the label.

Since we're talking about carbohydrates in this chapter, let's jump right to it on the label. The first line to look at is the one that says "Total Carbohydrate." This takes into account all of the various types of carbohydrates that are in this food and their quantities per serving. The types of carbohydrates that make up the total carbohydrate count are: dietary fiber, sugars, other carbohydrates, and sugar alcohols. These individual carbs might not be listed in the food label, but their presence is taken into consideration when calculating the total carbohydrate tally.

In our example on page 36, the Total Carbohydrate number is 24 grams. Remember, there are 4 calories/gram. That means that 96 calories per serving are coming from the carbohydrates. That's two-thirds of the total calories per serving of 130. Labels are not required to list all the types of carbohydrates in the food product; in fact, it's common for them to only list two or three. Our example lists two carbohydrate sources: dietary fiber (5 grams) and sugars (2 grams). That means of the 24 grams of carbohydrates in each serving, 7 grams come from dietary fiber and sugars. That means there are 17 grams of carbohydrates that are unaccounted for. These 17 grams are likely due to "other carbohydrates" and/or "sugar alcohols." The manufacturer doesn't give us the specifics about the source, but we can deduce that there are other carbohydrates beyond the dietary fiber and sugars, and thus the tally of 24 grams of total carbohydrate.

The sugars line deserves a closer inspection since this is one of those areas with which we need to concern ourselves when making a smart food choice. Unfortunately, manufacturers don't make it easy for the consumer to figure out the details of the type of sugars that are included in the food. Think for a moment. Why would manufacturers, whose financial success depends on your selecting their products, want to expose every grisly, calorie-laden, waistline-increasing, immune system–depressing detail about the unhealthy ingredients? The more you see behind the curtain, the more likely you are to pass on their product and choose the competitor's that's sitting on the shelf right next to it. So in the sugars section of the food label, you have no way of distinguishing between the natural sugars (found in many foods—fruit, vegetables, and dairy products) and the added sugars (found in snack foods—candy, baked goods, soda, etc.). But there is a way around this ambiguity. Look at the ingredient list and search for terms such as sugar, corn syrup or sweetener, dextrose, fructose, honey, and molasses to name just a few. If any of these items are high up on the ingredient list, then avoid them, since that means they are present in greater concentration. Remember, the ingredients are listed in descending order based on the amount the product contains.

Take a look at this nutrition label for one of America's favorite sugary snacks, Twinkies. This is what you'd find on the outside package of a ten-pack box. Note that each individual Twinkie is equivalent to a serving.

TWINKIES

Nutrition Facts

Serving Size: 1 Cake (43g)

Servings Per Container: 10

	Amount Per Serving	% Daily Value
Calories	150	
Calories from Fat	40	
Total Fat	4.5 g	7 %
Saturated Fat	2.5 g	13 %
Trans Fat	0 g	
Cholesterol	20 mg	7 %
Sodium	220 mg	9 %
Total Carbohydrate	27 g	9 %
Dietary Fiber	0 g	0 %
Sugars	18 g	
Protein	1 g	
	% Daily Value	
Vitamin A	0 %	
Vitamin C	0 %	
Calcium	0 %	
Iron	2 %	

You can see right away that there are 18 grams of sugar per serving. So where is this sugar coming from? Natural? Added? The nutritional facts on the label doesn't tell you; that's why we go to the next step and look at the ingredients.

Enriched Bleached Wheat Flour, Water, Sugar, Corn Syrup, High Fructose Corn Syrup, Partially Hydrogenated Vegetable and/or Animal Shortening, whole eggs, dextrose, contains 2% or less of: modified starch, glucose, leavenings, sweet dairy whey, soy protein isolate, calcium and sodium caseinate, soy flour, salt, mono and diglycerides, polysorbate 60, soy lecithin, cornstarch, cellulose gum, sodium stearoyl lactylate, natural and artificial flavors, sorbic acid, yellow 5, red 40. Contains wheat, egg, milk, and soybeans.

Your answer is right there in the first four lines. The sugars mentioned are: sugar, corn syrup, high fructose corn syrup, dextrose, starch, and glucose. This food product is *full* of added sugars. There is no mistaking them for the natural sugars that you might find in a pineapple or plum.

An important part of being able to detect those worthless added sugars is knowing all the names they can be called. No one ever said that food detective work was easy and straightforward, and for certain, manufacturers don't make it an easy task for you. But just by knowing the names you'll be able to root out almost all of the sugar compounds that are loaded into our foods and beverages.

Other Names for Added Sugars

Brown sugar	Invert sugar
Corn sweetener	Lactose
Corn syrup	Maltose
Dextrose	Malt syrup
Fructose	Molasses
Fruit juice blend	Raw sugar
Fruit juice concentrates	Sucrose
Glucose	Sugar
High fructose corn syrup	Syrup
Honey	

Now you are ready to start making smart choices about where you want your carbs to come from and how much you should consume. Carbs are the most abundant macronutrient in our food world, so get a handle on what's good and what's bad and learn to identify those hidden sugar sources. Here are some tips that you can apply right away as you leave carb hell and navigate your way into carb heaven.

Fat-Free Dangers

A common misperception is that when a label says "fat-free," it means that there aren't many calories or many sugars in the product. Wrong! In fact, one of the tricks that manufacturers use is to take the fat out of food so they can give it an appealing "fat-free" label, but then they replace or boost the sugar content of the food instead. The sugar replaces the taste that you typically lose when you take out the fat. This often means the calorie count is the same or even more than a full-fat product and the sugar count is equally alarming. The manufacturers are under no obligation to inform you of this substitution. They can make a claim that the food is 99 percent fat free and that's completely true. But the information they don't include in that eye-catching product name is what you need to find out on your own. Let's take a look at an example: a 6-ounce container of Yoplait 99% Fat-Free French Vanilla Yogurt. Sounds nice and healthy, right? Well, take a look at the label on the next page:

Nutrition Information

Serving Size: 6oz / 170g
Calories: 170
Calories from Fat: 15

Total Fat – Grams	1.5
% DV Fat	2
Saturated Fat – grams	1
% DV Saturated Fat	5
Trans Fat – grams	0
Cholesterol – mg	10
% DV Cholesterol	3
Sodium – mg	85
% DV Sodium	4
Potassium – mg	230
% DV Potassium	7
Total Carbohydrate – grams	33
% DV Carbohydrate	11
Dietary Fiber – grams	0
% DV Dietary Fiber	0
Sugars – grams	26
Protein – grams	5
% DV Protein	10
% DV Vitamin A	15
% DV Vitamin C	0
% DV Calcium	50
% DV Iron	4
% DV Vitamin D	50
% DV Phosphorus	0

Diet Exchanges
1 skim milk, 1-1/2 carbohydrate

This container of yogurt is 99 percent fat free but contains *170 calories*. How is this possible, considering that almost all of the fat is gone? Move down the list a little and the answer literally smacks you in the face. The Total Carbohydrate line says *33 grams*! That's right, 33 grams of carbohydrates of which *26 grams* are sugars! Ready for this? That's 6.2 teaspoons of sugar in that one serving of yogurt, almost the *entire* day's worth of added sugars that you should be consuming per the American Heart Association.

To drive home this point, let's look at Yoplait's 6-ounce Thick and Creamy Vanilla Yogurt. Here's the food label for this flavor. Unlike the

99 percent fat-free version, this product actually sounds like it's full of calories and other unhealthy ingredients. Let's take a quick look.

Nutrition Information

Serving Size: 6 oz / 170g
Calories: 180
Calories from Fat: 25

Total Fat – Grams	2.5
% DV Fat	4
Saturated Fat – grams	1.5
% DV Saturated Fat	8
Trans Fat – grams	0
Cholesterol – mg	15
% DV Cholesterol	4
Sodium – mg	110
% DV Sodium	5
Potassium – mg	290
% DV Potassium	8
Total Carbohydrate – grams	31
%DV Carbohydrate	10
Sugars – grams	28
Protein – grams	7
% DV Protein	13
% DV Vitamin A	15
% DV Calcium	30
% DV Vitamin D	20
% DV Phosphorus	20
Not a significant source of dietary fiber, vitamin C, or iron	

Diet Exchanges
1 skim milk, 1-1/2 carbohydrate, 1/2 fat

This product contains 180 calories, 31 grams of total carbohydrates of which 28 grams are sugar. This flavor surprisingly only has 10 more calories than the 99 percent fat free, which you would expect to have so much less. Also, the grams of sugar are almost the same, another surprise since you'd expect the thick and creamy version to be so much worse than the healthier-sounding 99 percent fat-free version.

The bottom line? Just because you see the words "fat free" or "99% fat free" in the name doesn't mean a product still doesn't have a significant amount of calories, and it definitely does not mean the sugar count is low. In many cases the sugar counts are actually higher than they are in a similar product that isn't fat free, and the calories are either close to being the same or slightly *increased*. Be a smart food detective and don't be fooled by tricky labeling!

Remember that carbs can be a good friend, but like any good friendship, you must respect them and not abuse them. Too many of us abuse carbs and that's when the relationship turns sour. Choose your carbs wisely and, as much as possible, avoid those that don't offer any nutritional value.

Tips for Adding Good Carbs to Your Diet

◆ Instead of snacking on chips and pretzels, try baby carrots, celery, or sliced cucumber. Dip them in peanut butter for some protein or sprinkle them with low-fat vinaigrette dressing for great taste with very few calories.

◆ Make it a goal to eat 2 servings of fruit each day. Eat at least one piece of fruit in the morning. For lunch or dinner slice an apple, pear, orange, or other fruit over your salad. Add half a cup of berries to your low-fat yogurt.

◆ Choose nuts and seeds occasionally for your snacks. Consume them in modest portions—a handful rather than the entire bag.

◆ Oatmeal, both old-fashioned and instant, is a great way to start the day. Mix in some bananas or berries and you will have provided your body with terrific fuel to propel you through the morning.

◆ Beans are your carb-healthy friends. Loaded with good carbs, beans also give you lots of protein and fiber.

◆ Top off your salads with chickpeas, lentils, or broccoli.

◆ Add vegetable purees to your soups, sauces, and casseroles.

EAT Plan

◆ Choose at least one dense carb with your meal. Whether it's a cup of brown rice, a cup of whole wheat pasta, or a couple of slices of 100% whole-grain bread, these options will fill you up on fewer calories and provide more nutrients than what you would get in white, refined foods.

◆ Dairy has its benefits, but make it healthier. Replace your typical fare with low-fat or skim milk, low-fat cheese, and fat-free yogurt. By the time you cook them into your food, you won't be able to taste the difference.

◆ Limit your consumption of cookies, cakes, doughnuts, and other refined sugar products to no more than 200 calories per day. If possible, stretch their frequency out even further to every other day. Replace these calories with sweet fruits.

The Whole Truth About Whole Grains

3

- ✦ The Whole-Grain Truth and Nothing but the Truth
- ✦ Your Best Whole-Grain Sources
- ✦ Whole Grains = Weight Loss
- ✦ Beware of Whole-Grain Imposters

You'd have to have been living in a deep fryer for most of your life not to know that whole grains are good for your health. Food manufacturers have been bombarding you with this information through heavy advertising, and food experts have been on every morning news show extolling the health benefits of whole-grain products. This is one of those rare examples where you *can* believe the hype. Whole-grain foods are some of the healthiest in the world and it all comes down to a seed.

What Is a Whole Grain?

A grain is a small, dry, hard seed harvested from crops of grasses, among which are wheat, corn, rye, oats, rice, and millet. Whole grains contain all three parts of the grain: the bran, the endosperm, and the germ.

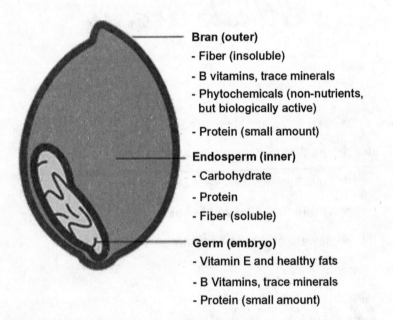

Bran (outer)
- Fiber (insoluble)
- B vitamins, trace minerals
- Phytochemicals (non-nutrients, but biologically active)
- Protein (small amount)

Endosperm (inner)
- Carbohydrate
- Protein
- Fiber (soluble)

Germ (embryo)
- Vitamin E and healthy fats
- B Vitamins, trace minerals
- Protein (small amount)

The *bran* is the multilayered outer skin of the grain that serves as a protector of the other two parts—the endosperm and germ. Sunlight, pests, water, and disease are kept out of the kernel by this tough protective coat that also contains important B vitamins, antioxidants, and fiber.

The *endosperm* is the food supply for the germ. It provides essential energy to the young plant so it can send roots down into the ground to absorb water and nutrients as well as send sprouts up in the air to capture the sunlight and harness its photosynthesizing power (the process of using sunlight to make carbohydrates in plants). This is the largest part of the grain. It contains starchy carbohydrates, proteins, and only small amounts of vitamins and minerals.

The *germ* is the grain's reproductive component—the embryo. If it's fertilized by pollen, it will sprout into a new plant. The germ contains many B vitamins, some protein, minerals, and healthy fats.

Think of whole grains as the purest form of grain in which the unit has been left intact and all of its great nutrients are available to us when we eat them. Now imagine taking this grain and smashing it into countless pieces. This is what happens when grains are put through a grinder to mechanically remove the bran and endosperm, a process that you might hear referred to as "milling." And voilà, this is how we arrive at another important term you've probably heard a million times: *refined grain.*

From a nutritional standpoint, refined grains are like cheap knockoffs of expensive handbags. They are a fraction of the cost, can be found all over the place, and may look like the real thing at first until you start noticing the defects and imperfections. Refining grains converts whole grains into white flour. With the removal of the bran and germ, the refined white flour loses all but a small fraction of its original nutrition, causing almost a total loss of fiber, a 25 percent loss of the grain's protein, and the loss of seventeen or more other key nutrients. Now you can understand why nutritionists are constantly trying to get us to eat whole-grain bread instead of white bread. Whole-grain bread is overwhelmingly superior.

So if refined grains are so nutritionally inferior, why would someone create them? Like most things when it comes to business: it's all about money. By removing the tough bran coat and germ, the grains now have a softer, finer texture that's more attractive to the consumer, making the food less expensive and improving how long these products can live on the shelf. The longer it takes for a product to spoil, the more time the grocery store owner has to sell it to you, and the less spoiled food has to be thrown away, thereby increasing the store's profits.

Our last important concept is that of a food being *enriched* (which translates to "medium good"). Most refined grains are enriched, which means that after many of the vitamins and nutrients have been lost in the refining process, certain B vitamins (thiamin, riboflavin, niacin, folic acid) and iron are added back after the processing has occurred. It's important to note, however, that fiber is not added back during the enriching process.

Common Whole-Grain Food Products

The interest in whole-grain products has risen dramatically over the last several years and experts forecast this interest will only grow. As consumers become more aware of the nutritional benefits of whole grains, they are choosing these products over their refined counterparts. According to a report from the consumer market research firm Packaged Facts entitled *The U.S. Market for Whole and Other Grains: Trends and Developments,* retail sales of whole grains in 2008 were estimated to be $5 billion. This was a dramatic increase of 17 percent over the previous year.

Hundreds of millions of whole-grain products line the shelves of our grocery stores as manufacturers have responded to the growing consumer demand for healthier grains. With so many products making so many claims, it's not always easy to distinguish what's real and what isn't (more on this later), but knowing some of the whole grains out there is a good start. Below is a quick reference guide to some of the common and less common whole grains that you'll find at the market.

Common Whole Grains

Brown rice	Popcorn
Wild rice	Whole oats
Whole wheat	Buckwheat
Barley	Flaxseed
Oatmeal	Corn grits (not instant)
Whole rye	Couscous
Bulgur	

Less Common Whole Grains

Quinoa	Spelt
Millet	Wheatberries
Amaranth	Cracked wheat
Sorghum	Farro
Triticale	

Breakfast cereals can be a good and convenient source of whole grains. They are also an easy way to get started on meeting your daily whole-grain recommended intake. But there are so many cereals on the market using so many different phrases to describe their contents that it's confusing when trying to determine the best sources for whole grains. The simple chart on page 52 can help you make the smartest choices in the morning.

Cold Cereals		Hot Cereals	
Whole Grain	**Mostly Refined Grain**	**Whole Grain**	**Mostly Refined Grain**
Cheerios	Basic 4	Oat Bran	Cream of Rice
Granola or muesli	Corn Flakes	Oatmeal	Cream of Wheat
Grape-Nuts	Frosted Flakes	Quaker Multigrain	Grits
Nutri-Grain	Just Right	Ralston High Fiber	
Raisin Bran	Kix, Corn Pops	Roman Meal	
Shredded Wheat	Product 19	Wheatena	
Total	Puffed Wheat	Bob's Red Mill	
Wheat Germ	Rice Krispies	Kashi GOLEAN	
Wheaties	Special K		
Life	Apple Jacks		
Kashi	Cap'n Crunch		
Golden Grahams	Cocoa Puffs		
Wheat Chex	Lucky Charms		
Multi-Bran Chex	Puffed Rice		
	Special K		

Partial Source: Center for Science in the Public Interest

How Many Whole Grains Should We Eat Each Day

The USDA recommends that we consume three servings of whole grains each day. Unfortunately, several studies have shown that we fall far below this target, especially when it comes to our teens and young adults. In a recent study, researchers from the University of Minnesota

School of Public Health reported that young people are consuming less than one serving of whole grains per day.[1]

So what does a serving of whole grains look like? It's actually quite simple to tell. Below you'll find several examples that will help you in your effort to know just how many servings of whole grains you're consuming. Also, look at the food label on the package; often manufacturers will tell you how many servings of whole grains are contained in each serving of their product.

A Serving of Whole Grains

$1/2$ cup cooked brown rice or other cooked grain

$1/2$ cup cooked hot cereal, such as oatmeal

1 slice 100% whole-grain bread

1 very small (30 grams or 1 ounce) 100% whole-grain muffin

1 cup 100% whole-grain ready-to-eat cereal

1 ounce uncooked 100% whole-grain pasta, brown rice, or other grain

$1/2$ cup cooked whole-grain pasta

2 small pancakes made with whole-grain flour

1 small waffle made with whole-grain flour

1 small muffin made with whole-grain flour

1 flat whole wheat tortilla (6-inch diameter)

2 cups plain popcorn

1 small (35 grams) whole wheat waffle

Sources: Whole Grain Council, USDA Food Pyramid, Canada's Food Guide

Health Benefits of Whole Grains

Whole grains are some of the most nutritious foods in our diet. They are typically low in fat, contain little or no cholesterol, and are

full of vitamins, minerals, and other nutrients that have a tremendously positive impact on our health. Whole grains are also rich in
complex carbohydrates—the good carbs—which are also an important
component of a healthy diet. Whether it's fiber, vitamin E, selenium,
zinc, copper, or iron, whole grains supply disease-fighting nutrients
that can reduce some of the effects of aging and, according to some
studies, help to bolster our immune system. Below are some of the
health benefits associated with a diet rich in whole grains. It's because
of this vast array of benefits that health advocates recommend loading
up on whole grains and reducing consumption of the less nutritious
refined grains.

Health Benefits of Whole Grains

- Substantially lower type 2 diabetes risk

- Help avoid gallstones

- Reduce risks of heart disease

- Reduce risk of stroke

- Reduce risk of cancer

- Lower risk of obesity

- Reduce risk of high blood pressure

- Lower risk of colon cancer

- Slow the buildup of dangerous plaque in arteries

Whole Grains and Weight Loss

Beyond the commonly known health benefits of whole grains, experienced dieters and nutritionists are also aware of their contribu-

tions to weight loss. There are four major ways in which they can help you shed those extra pounds. First, whole grains are typically higher in protein content compared to their counterparts that have undergone the refinement process. There is plenty of evidence that increasing the amount of protein-rich foods you consume will help with weight loss. Proteins require more energy to digest, and therefore cause the body to burn more calories. Research has also shown that diets higher in protein and moderate in carbs, along with regular exercise, can reduce fats in the blood and maintain lean muscle mass while burning fat to fuel the body.

Whole grains are also low on the glycemic index (GI). Go back to page 22 for the full discussion of the glycemic index, but the simplified explanation is that the GI is a function of how quickly a particular food is broken down by the body and enters the bloodstream. The GI is a measure of how fast and how high the body experiences this rise or spike in the blood sugar level. Changes in blood sugar are part of the process of determining hunger and appetite. If the food you're consuming is used up by the body quickly, then it follows that you will feel hungry sooner than you would if you consumed food that took longer for the body to process. Eating whole grains and other low GI foods stabilizes your blood sugar levels so that throughout the day they change gradually rather than the spiking that's seen with refined foods and those high in sugars.

The fiber found in whole grains is another advantage in weight loss. You can fill yourself up with less food and thus consume fewer calories overall. Fiber has many health benefits, including slowing the speed at which our digestive tract breaks down food, which in effect makes you feel full longer. The longer you feel full, the less urge you'll have to eat and the fewer calories you'll consume.

Lastly, the fiber in whole grains can help decrease how much fat is absorbed by the body. Fiber can increase how fast stool moves through the digestive tract and thus affect how often you go to the bathroom. The faster your body gets rid of waste, the less time there is for the body to absorb fat and other high-calorie substances.

How to Know If Food Really Is Made of Whole Grains

Manufacturers are fully aware of the health benefits of whole grains and the level of quality they bring to a food product. They also know that in a health-conscious society, more consumers are becoming more discriminating about what they eat. The smart eater is also a smart shopper and will spend an extra few minutes looking at the food label to make sure they're choosing a product with the most to offer. This is why it's to your advantage to be a food detective when walking down the grocery store aisles. Don't forget that the food industry is an extremely competitive marketplace with trillions of dollars at stake. Manufacturers are in a daily fight in a very limited store space to attract you to their product in an effort to convince you to choose theirs over a competitor's. Unfortunately, this means there is often a lot of gamesmanship when it comes to marketing products and the wording that's put on the packaging. Because whole-grain products are the "healthier" products and the demand for them is continually increasing as consumers learn more about their benefits, food manufacturers sometimes play tricks to make you think their products contain more of the "good stuff," when actually they don't.

You will come across several words or phases that look impressive, but don't really tell the entire story, for example: "multigrain," "whole-grain blend," "made with whole grain," "100% wheat," or "stone ground." Multigrain simply means that the product contains more than one kind of grain. This, however, doesn't mean they contain *whole* grains. And if a product with this labeling does contain whole grains, there's no guarantee it actually contains much.

The phrase "100% wheat" is really tricky. Many people mistakenly believe this is another way of saying whole grain, but it's not. To say "100% wheat" simply means that the only grain contained in the product is wheat. It does not mean the wheat is whole. It could be refined, which means the nutritious parts have been stripped away. The phrase that you should be looking for is "100% *whole* wheat."

To help consumers more accurately identify true whole grains, the Whole Grains Council has created an official packaging symbol that you can find easily. This Whole Grain Stamp started to appear in mid-2005 and has become increasingly more common. The stamp on a package has become a convenient guarantee that the food inside contains real whole grains. There are two types of stamps, one that is considered the basic stamp and one that is marked "100% whole grain." The basic stamp appears on products containing at least half a serving of whole grain per labeled serving—that would be 8 grams per serving. The 100% stamp assures you that the food contains a full serving or more of whole grain in each labeled serving (16 grams), and that *all* the grain is whole grain. This labeling makes it much easier when you're trying to meet the recommended three-servings per day of whole grains—48 grams in total.

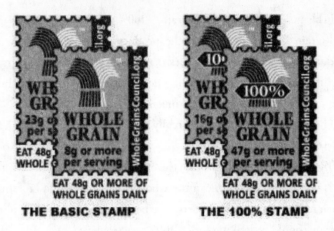

THE BASIC STAMP   **THE 100% STAMP**

Just because a food package doesn't have the whole-grain stamp, however, doesn't mean there aren't whole grains in it. While many whole-grain products have this stamp, not all of them do since using it is voluntary. So you still need another method to find out if the food is the real deal. If you see the following words on the package, then you know the food contains all parts of the grain and you're getting all the nutrients of the whole grain:

Whole grain

Whole wheat

Stoneground whole grain

Brown rice

Oats, oatmeal (including old-fashioned oatmeal, instant)

Wheatberries

Sometimes the whole grain is partially refined, so some of the parts of the grain might be missing. This means it's likely you are not getting the full benefit of the whole grain. Products labeled with the following phrases fit into this category:

Wheat flour
Semolina
Durum wheat
Organic flour
Multigrain

There are some words that look like they are describing a healthy whole grain when in actuality they *never* describe whole grains. They are still healthier than the alternatives of refined and processed foods, but they just aren't considered to be the superstars whole grains are. The following fit into this category:

Enriched flour
Degerminated
Bran
Wheat germ

The last tip in detecting real whole grains is to read the list of ingredients. Typically the ingredients are listed in descending order based on how much of them is contained within the food. Make note of the first ingredient listed, since that is what predominates. As an example, look at two Pepperidge Farm breads—white bread and 100% whole wheat bread. This is the list of ingredients for the white bread:

UNBROMATED UNBLEACHED ENRICHED WHEAT FLOUR, MALTED BARLEY FLOUR, NIACIN, REDUCED IRON, THIAMIN MONONITRATE

(VITAMIN B1), RIBOFLAVIN (VITAMIN B2), FOLIC ACID], WATER, HIGH
FRUCTOSE CORN SYRUP, SOYBEAN OIL, YEAST, CONTAINS 2 PERCENT
OR LESS OF: SALT, CALCIUM PROPIONATE (TO RETARD SPOILAGE),
VEGETABLE MONOGLYCERIDES, CALCIUM CARBONATE, NONFAT MILK,
ENZYMES, BUTTER AND HONEY

Notice that the first ingredient is wheat flour. It's not *whole* wheat flour,
but simply wheat flour. It is not made from whole grains, but rather grains
that have been refined and stripped of their good nutrients. Notice another word that comes before wheat flour—"enriched." This is a word
that you will see often and you should know what it means. Wheat flour
is made when the whole wheat grain is ground and then refined (processed) to give the bread a finer texture. Remember, when the whole grain
is refined, the bran and germ are stripped away, which causes the food to
lose most of its nutrients. In an effort to make the flour healthier, *some*
nutrients—thiamin, riboflavin, and niacin—are added back. But the en-
richment is not perfect and there are nutrients such as fiber that are lost
forever in the refining process. So, enriched flour is certainly not "whole"
flour, but it is healthier than the processed flour that hasn't been enriched.

Now let's take a look at the ingredients of Pepperidge Farm's 100%
whole wheat bread:

WHOLE WHEAT FLOUR, WATER, HIGH FRUCTOSE CORN SYRUP, WHEAT
GLUTEN, SOYBEAN OIL, YEAST, UNSULPHURED MOLASSES, CON-
TAINS 2% OR LESS OF OAT FIBER, HONEY, SALT, CALCIUM PROPIO-
NATE (TO RETARD SPOILAGE), MONOGLYCERIDES, NONFAT MILK,
BUTTER, SOY LECITHIN AND ENZYMES

Notice that the first ingredient is "whole wheat flour." This tells us two
important things. First, it tells us that whole wheat flour is the major

ingredient. Second, the word "whole" in front of it tells you that it's made from real whole grain and that the nutrients have not been stripped away as in the previous example of the white bread. High fructose corn syrup is also high on the list, so if you're trying to reduce your consumption of this ingredient, then you might consider looking for a whole grain bread that doesn't contain it or has it much lower on the list.

There are plenty of authentic whole-grain products in grocery stores, but it's important not to confuse them with the whole-grain imposters. You are now armed with enough information about whole grains and refined grains to make smart choices. Switching to whole grains and cutting back on the refined foods is a small change that can deliver amazing results. It won't take long before you start noticing the healthy impact these nutrient-rich whole grains can deliver.

6 Recommended Whole-Grain Products

Lundberg Rice Blends

Original Wheetabix Cereal

Wasa Crispbread

Ezekiel breads, rolls, pasta

Hodgson Mill Pancake/Waffle Mix, pasta, and other products

Earth's Best Cereals and Snacks for Children

Tips for Adding Whole Grains to Your Diet

◆ Enjoy breakfasts that include high-fiber cereals, such as bran flakes, shredded wheat, or oatmeal.

◆ Substitute half the white flour with whole wheat flour in your recipes for cookies, muffins, quick breads, and pancakes.

◆ Substitute whole wheat toast or whole-grain bagels for plain bagels. Substitute low-fat bran muffins for pastries.

◆ Add half a cup of cooked bulgur, wild rice, or barley to bread stuffing.

◆ Make sandwiches using whole-grain breads or rolls. Swap out white-flour tortillas with whole wheat versions.

◆ Add half a cup of cooked wheat or rye berries, wild rice, brown rice, or barley to your soup, whether it's canned or homemade.

◆ Replace white rice with kasha, brown rice, wild rice, or bulgur.

◆ Use whole cornmeal for corn cakes, corn breads, and corn muffins.

◆ Feature wild rice or barley in soups, stews, casseroles, and salads.

◆ Add a handful of oats to your yogurt.

◆ Add whole grains, such as cooked brown rice or whole-grain bread crumbs, to ground meat or poultry for extra body.

◆ Look for cereal made with grains like kamut, kasha (buckwheat), or spelt.

◆ Use rolled oats or crushed bran cereal in recipes instead of dry bread crumbs.

Whole Grains: Cooking Tips

1. Rinse: Just prior to cooking, rinse whole grains thoroughly in cold water until the water runs clear, then strain them to remove any dirt or debris.

2. Cook: As a general rule, you can cook whole grains by simply adding the grain to boiling water, return water to a boil, then simmer, covered, until tender. Cooking hint: Use broth instead of water for even more flavor.

3. Test: Just like pasta, always test whole grains for doneness before taking them off the heat; most whole grains should be slightly chewy when cooked.

4. Fluff: When grains are done, remove them from the heat and gently fluff them with a fork. Then cover them and set aside to let sit for 5 to 10 minutes and serve.

Source: *Whole Food Markets*

EAT Plan

✦ Try to consume 3 servings (16 grams = 1 serving) of whole grains every other day. Increase your consumption to reach the ultimate goal of 3 servings of whole grains every day.

✦ No more white breads. Switch to whole-grain breads. If you want the softer texture of white breads and don't want the hardness of the whole grains, then you can get 100% whole wheat breads that are labeled soft (the grain is ground more). This is like eating white bread, but instead it's made from whole grains and has all the nutrients still in it.

✦ Start your day with at least one serving of whole grains. Whole-grain cereals are convenient, or try a whole-grain muffin or whole-grain pancakes.

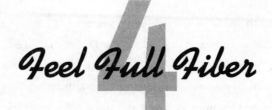

Feel Full Fiber

- ✦ We Require Fiber
- ✦ Fill Up with Fiber
- ✦ The Magic of Fiber
- ✦ Quick and Easy Fiber Chart of Foods

*F*iber is a word you've heard a thousand times, but one whose definition you might not understand very well. The reason why so many people don't know what fiber is and what it does is not because it's a complicated subject. Just the opposite is true. The world of fiber is a relatively simple one to comprehend, but the reason why knowledge of this nutrient is elusive for so many is because few people take the time to explain what fiber is, where it comes from, and what it does to promote good health. People who have a working knowledge of this microscopic plant part are much better for it as they can now incorporate it correctly in their diets and enjoy the long list of benefits it offers.

Let's get the basic definition under our belts. There are two main classes of carbohydrates: starch, which our bodies can digest, and fiber, which our bodies are not able to digest. Fiber is mainly found in the outer layers of all plants that are eaten for food, including fruits, vegetables, grains, and legumes (beans, peas, lentils), but is never found in animals. Now, all fiber is not the same. There are two major types of fiber: soluble and insoluble. Soluble fiber dissolves in water to form a gel-like substance. Insoluble fiber passes though our digestive system almost intact because we can't break it down. It increases the movement of material through the digestive system, adding bulk to our stool, and acting as a sponge to absorb water. The total fiber content of a food is considered to be the amount of soluble fiber contained within the food added to the amount of insoluble fiber. We should consume both in a healthy diet.

Common Sources of Soluble Fiber

Oats	Strawberries
Legumes (beans, peas, and soybeans)	Blueberries
	Bananas
Apples	Nuts and seeds
Pears	Lentils

Common Sources of Insoluble Fiber

Whole wheat foods	Carrots
Barley	Cucumbers
Couscous	Zucchini
Brown rice	Celery
Bulgur	Tomato
Seeds	Wheat bran

Source: Harvard School of Public Health

How Much Fiber Do You Need?

To say that Americans don't get enough fiber in their diets is an understatement. Every major study shows that our fiber consumption falls embarrassingly short of national recommendations as well as the amount consumed in other countries. The American Dietetic Association recommends that we consume 20 to 35 grams of fiber each day, but the average American eats only 15 grams per day, not even coming close to the lower limit of what's recommended. By comparison, people in China consume as much as 77 grams of fiber per day, one reason experts believe they have significantly lower rates of colon cancer (more on this later).

The general rule is that the more calories you eat each day, the more fiber you need. The Institute of Medicine recommends that children and adults consume 14 grams of fiber for every 1,000 calories of food they eat each day. What would this look like? Let's say you consume 2,500 calories per day. You should then also be consuming 35 grams of fiber on a daily basis. A person who consumes 1,500 calories should be taking in 21 grams of fiber. The following chart can help you determine the amount of fiber you should consume. If you consume more or fewer calories than the averages that are listed in the chart, then adjust your fiber consumption accordingly. If you're unsure how many calories you eat each day, know that you should be eating *at least* 20 grams of fiber per day.

Daily Fiber Requirement		
Age (Years)	**Average Daily Calories Consumed**	**Fiber Intake (Grams)**
Children		
1–3	1,404	19
4–8	1,789	25

continued

Age (Years)	Average Daily Calories Consumed	Fiber Intake (Grams)
Boys and Men		
9–13	2,265	31
14–18	2,840	38
19–30	2,818	38
31–50	2,554	38
51–70	2,162	30
70+	1,821	30
Girls and Women		
9–13	1,910	26
14–18	1,901	26
19–30	1,791	25
31–50	1,694	25
51–70	1,536	21
70+	1,381	21

Source: Institute of Medicine. *Dietary Reference Intakes for Energy, Carbohydrate, Fiber, Fat, Fatty Acids, Cholesterol, Protein, and Amino Acids.* Washington, D.C.: The National Academies Press, 2002. Retrieved from http://books.nap.edu/openbook.php?isbn= 0309085373.

Consuming 20 grams of fiber per day is a minimum requirement. The following are a couple of examples that show that meeting this requirement isn't very difficult.

1 cup of raspberries as part of your breakfast: 8.3 grams of fiber/ 60 calories

1 cup of lentil soup for lunch: 15.6 grams of fiber/230 calories

Total fiber intake: 23.9 grams and just 290 calories

1 cup of strawberries with your breakfast: 3.3 grams of fiber/
   43 calories

1 cup of green peas at lunch: 8.8 grams of fiber/134 calories

1 cup of carrots at lunch: 3.7 grams of fiber/53 calories

1 cup of collard greens with your dinner: 5.3 grams of fiber/49
   calories

Total fiber intake: 21.1 grams and just 279 calories

The Magical Benefits of Fiber

Only if you've been living under a rock in the middle of a desert for the last twenty years would it be possible for you not to have heard or read that fiber is good for you. Every major organization, from the American Dietetic Association to the American Heart Association, has sung the praises of including more fiber in our diets. Large, credible studies have shown that fiber can be extremely helpful in lowering the risks of developing a broad spectrum of diseases. Let's start with the heart first, since diseases of this organ system are the number one killer in the United States.

Fiber and Cardiovascular Disease

Along with exercise, one of the best things you can do to protect your heart is to follow a diet high in fiber. There have been many studies that support this finding. Researchers in a Harvard study of over 40,000 male health professionals found that a high total dietary fiber intake was linked to a 40 percent lower risk of coronary heart disease compared to a low fiber intake.[1]

In another major study involving more than 34,000 people, researchers found that there was a 44 percent reduced risk of nonfatal coronary heart disease and an 11 percent reduced risk of fatal coronary heart disease for those who ate whole wheat bread compared to those who ate white bread.[2]

Fiber has also been shown to reduce the risk of developing metabolic syndrome, a group of factors (high blood pressure, high insulin resistance, excess weight, high levels of triglycerides, and low levels of HDL [good] cholesterol) that can increase the chances of developing heart disease and diabetes. Several studies show that increasing your intake of breakfast cereal fiber and whole grains can reduce the risk factors that lead to this syndrome.

Then there's the dreaded LDL, or "bad cholesterol," that can cause plaque to build up in your arteries and lead to heart attacks and strokes. According to an analysis of several studies, soluble fiber has been shown to modestly reduce bad cholesterol levels better than if one were to simply eat a diet low in saturated and trans fats and cholesterol alone.[3] When you look at grains, for example, oats contain the highest proportion of soluble fiber.

Fiber and Diabetes

Several studies have examined the role of fiber in the development of diabetes. The good news is that researchers have found that fiber helps to reduce the risk of developing type 2 diabetes. The type of fiber that seems to have the greatest effect is the soluble variety, which also happens to be the fiber most commonly found in breakfast cereal. Fiber has also been shown to be beneficial for people who already have diabetes. Controlling blood sugar levels is critical for the long-term health of diabetics and to prevent them from developing debilitating and sometimes dangerous complications such as heart disease, eye disease, kidney disease, and neurologic problems. Soluble fiber is believed to help reduce the absorption of the sugar glucose in the stomach, thus reducing its level in the blood. Insoluble fiber is believed to also help the cause further down in the digestive tract by increasing the speed that sugars pass through the intestines, thus decreasing their absorption into the bloodstream.[4]

Fiber and Weight Loss

Several studies have looked at fiber and its impact on weight loss. The research overwhelmingly shows that fiber can be helpful for any program in which you are trying to lose weight or avoid gaining weight. There are several ways in which fiber delivers this benefit. First, fiber typically causes you to eat more slowly as it requires more time to chew. Increasing the amount of time you spend consuming a meal gives the body more time to recognize when your appetite is satisfied, thus sending an efficient signal to stop eating, which ultimately can prevent overeating.

Fiber is believed to increase the amount of time that food stays in the stomach. This means that your stomach is stretched for a longer period of time and experiences a feeling of fullness longer than if the stomach had emptied the food more quickly.

Fiber is also known for its low energy density, or how many calories there are within a certain amount of food. For example, one bacon cheeseburger has a relatively high energy density, delivering as many as 600 calories or more. A lower energy density meal might be a roast turkey breast sandwich (3 ounces) on whole wheat bread with low-fat cheese (1 ounce), lettuce and tomatoes along with a medium apple, several celery sticks, a cup of vegetable soup, whole-grain crackers, and a glass of water. All that food contains only 545 calories. Fiber is helpful in weight loss because it allows you to increase the volume of what you're eating and feel full on fewer calories.

Fiber and Bowel Movements

Fiber delivers some of its greatest benefits to our gastrointestinal tract and the process of forming stool. Fiber binds water, which gives the stool greater bulk. The water also softens the stool, which allows it to move more easily and without pain within the digestive tract. For someone suffering from constipation, fiber can be helpful in increasing the number of bowel movements each day and improving the ease of the stool's passing. The best relief is likely to be found with a combination of soluble and insoluble fiber rather than just the soluble fiber commonly found in the over-the-counter supplements on its own. Just make sure that when you increase your fiber intake to help your bowel movements that you also increase the amount of water you consume, or the fiber will have an effect you don't want—making the stool hard and difficult to pass.

Fiber and Colon Cancer

There has been a lot of discussion about whether a diet rich in fiber can help reduce the risk of colon cancer. Unfortunately, like many issues in medical science, there is no unanimous opinion one way or the other. Some researchers look at the anecdotal evidence to support their theory that fiber decreases the risk of developing colon cancer. They point to the Chinese, who consume on average double or more the fiber that Americans and other Westerners do. The Chinese also have tremendously lower rates of colon cancer when compared to Americans, and many believe that it's the high-fiber, low-fat quality of their diet that's making the difference.

There is, however, a mound of scientific evidence to the contrary. Large, well-designed studies have for the most part failed to show a link between fiber and colon cancer. One famous Harvard study followed 80,000 nurses for sixteen years and found that there wasn't any strong association between dietary fiber intake and the risk for either colon cancer or the precursors to colon cancer—polyps.[5]

While this conflicting evidence doesn't give us a clear answer about fiber's relationship to colon cancer, there is enough evidence about fiber's other benefits for us to continue to recommend it. Some experts have also speculated that people who eat foods higher in fiber (i.e., fruits, vegetables, and whole grains) are likely to have a healthier overall lifestyle and a better quality of life.

How Much Fiber Is in Your Food?

It's not always easy to tell exactly how much fiber is contained in the food you eat. Sometimes the food labels on the packaging will list fiber and the amount that is contained in each serving of the food product, but often you won't get this important information. To give you an idea of how much fiber some common foods contain, refer to the chart below.

Food Item	Serving Size	Total Fiber/ Serving (g)	Soluble Fiber/ Serving (g)	Insoluble Fiber/ Serving (g)
Vegetables, Cooked				
Asparagus	½ cup	2.8	1.7	1.1
Beets, flesh only	½ cup	1.8	0.8	1.0
Broccoli	½ cup	2.4	1.2	1.2
Brussels sprouts	½ cup	3.8	2.0	1.8
Corn, whole kernel, canned	½ cup	1.6	0.2	1.4
Carrots, sliced	½ cup	2.0	1.1	0.9
Cauliflower	½ cup	1.0	0.4	0.6

continued

Food Item	Serving Size	Total Fiber/ Serving (g)	Soluble Fiber/ Serving (g)	Insoluble Fiber/ Serving (g)
Vegetables, Cooked				
Green beans, canned	1/2 cup	2.0	0.5	1.5
Kale	1/2 cup	2.5	0.7	1.8
Okra, frozen	1/2 cup	4.1	1.0	3.1
Peas, green, frozen	1/2 cup	4.3	1.3	3.0
Potato, sweet, flesh only	1/2 cup	4.0	1.8	2.2
Spinach	1/2 cup	1.6	0.5	1.1
Tomato sauce	1/2 cup	1.7	0.8	0.9
Turnip	1/2 cup	4.8	1.7	3.1
Raw Vegetables				
Cabbage, red	1 cup	1.5	0.6	0.9
Carrots, fresh	1, 7 1/2" long	2.3	1.1	1.2
Celery, fresh	1 cup chopped	1.7	0.7	1.0
Cucumber, fresh	1 cup	0.5	0.2	0.3
Lettuce, iceberg	1 cup	0.5	0.1	0.4
Mushrooms, fresh	1 cup pieces	0.8	0.1	0.7
Onion, fresh	1/2 cup chopped	1.7	0.9	0.8
Pepper, green, fresh	1 cup chopped	1.7	0.7	1.0
Tomato, fresh	1 medium	1.0	0.1	0.9
Fruits				
Apple, red, fresh w/skin	1 small	2.8	1.0	1.8
Applesauce, canned	1/2 cup	2.0	0.7	1.3
Apricots, dried	7 halves	2.0	1.1	0.9
Apricots, fresh w/skin	4	3.5	1.8	1.7
Banana, fresh	1/2 small	1.1	0.3	0.8
Blueberries, fresh	3/4 cup	1.4	0.3	1.1

Food Item	Serving Size	Total Fiber/ Serving (g)	Soluble Fiber/ Serving (g)	Insoluble Fiber/ Serving (g)
Fruits				
Cherries, black, fresh	12 large	1.3	0.6	0.7
Figs, dried	1½	3.0	1.4	1.6
Grapefruit, fresh	½ medium	1.6	1.1	0.5
Grapes, fresh w/skin	15 small	0.5	0.2	0.3
Kiwifruit, fresh, flesh only	1 large	1.7	0.7	1.0
Mango, fresh, flesh only	½ small	2.9	1.7	1.2
Melon, cantaloupe	1 cup cubed	1.1	0.3	0.8
Orange, fresh, flesh only	1 small	2.9	1.8	1.1
Peach, fresh, w/skin	1 medium	2.0	1.0	1.0
Pear, fresh, w/skin	½ large	2.9	1.1	1.8
Plum, red, fresh	2 medium	2.4	1.1	1.3
Prunes, dried	3 medium	1.7	1.0	0.7
Raisins, dried	2 Tbsp.	0.4	0.2	0.2
Raspberries, fresh	1 cup	3.3	0.9	2.4
Strawberries, fresh	1¼ cups	2.8	1.1	1.7
Watermelon	1¼ cups cubed	0.6	0.4	0.2

Simple Tips to Add Fiber to Your Diet

✦ Snack on raw vegetables such as carrots, celery, and cucumbers instead of chips, crackers, or candy.

✦ Replace white rice, bread, and pasta with brown rice and whole-grain foods.

✦ Instead of putting meat in your chili or soups, add legumes (peas, beans, lentils) or you can keep ½ the meat and replace the other ½ with legumes.

✦ Replace sugar-coated morning cereals with whole-grain cereals.

✦ Eat whole fruits instead of drinking fruit juices—the fiber's in the skin.

✦ Increase your fiber consumption slowly over 2 to 3 weeks to give your body time to adjust.

✦ Add flaxseeds, seeds, or nuts to your salad, soup, yogurt, or cereal.

✦ Add beans or peas to your salad or soup.

✦ Stock your freezer with frozen fruits such as blueberries, strawberries, and raspberries—add these to your cereal, shakes, or yogurt.

Too Much Fiber

While fiber is important for a healthy diet, like many other things in life, there can be too much of a good thing. Since fiber carries water out of the body, consuming too much can lead to dehydration, intestinal cramping and discomfort, bloating, and excess gas. This is why consuming large amounts of fiber means also needing to consume large amounts of water.

Fiber speeds the movement of foods through our digestive tract. This can be a good thing, but if the food moves too fast for too long, it can have negative consequences, since it reduces the amount of time the body has to absorb the food's nutrients. Reduced absorption of these important minerals such as iron, zinc, magnesium, and calcium can cause deficiencies that if not monitored or corrected can negatively impact your health.

To make sure you get the most benefits out of your fiber, be careful to increase your fiber consumption slowly over 2 to 3 weeks to give your body time to adjust. Make sure you drink plenty of water every day—at least 6 glasses or more.

Fiber Supplements

Some people, regardless of how hard they try, won't consume enough fiber. Many will turn to supplements—fiber in a pill or a powder—to make up for what they're not able to get in food. Before you use any supplement, you should check with your healthcare provider to make sure that it's safe and right for you. Supplements, unlike prescription drugs, are not approved or monitored by the U.S. Food and Drug Administration (FDA). There is relatively little oversight of the supplements market, which means that manufacturers are largely free to manufacture and market their products without having to submit credible research-based evidence of their products' safety and effectiveness. The lack of oversight of the supplements market is a big issue, but the relevant point here is that if you plan on taking a supplement, get an unbiased and professional opinion.

Regardless of what advertising says about supplements, you should know that the best source of fiber is in food. Supplements are acceptable in an emergency situation or if you simply can't get enough via your food in any particular week, but the number one choice is dietary. Supplements typically supply only a very restricted type of fiber and not much else. Meeting your fiber requirements by making smart food choices also means you'll be eating vitamins, minerals, and other nutrients that are typically contained in fiber-rich foods.

EAT Plan

✦ Consume the appropriate amount of fiber each day based on your gender and age. Refer to the table located in the beginning of this chapter.

✦ Choose those fruits and vegetables that deliver the strongest fiber punch: high-fiber cereals, wheat bran, split peas, lentils, kidney beans, black beans, chickpeas (garbanzo beans), lima beans, navy beans, raspberries, apples (with skin), pears (with skin), strawberries, bananas, and oranges.

✦ If you are a cereal eater, make sure that at least every other day you eat a whole-grain cereal.

Protein Bonanza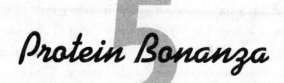

- ✦ The Pros of Protein
- ✦ The Building Blocks of Life
- ✦ All Proteins Aren't Equal
- ✦ Your Best Sources of Protein

*P*roteins are everywhere. Literally. In our bodies, in our food, in animals—proteins are one of the most important compounds in the world. Without proteins we couldn't live. Just as consuming carbohydrates and fats is critical to a healthy diet, so is consuming the right type and quantity of proteins. Protein, just like fats and carbohydrates, is considered to be a *macronutrient,* because the body needs a relatively large amount of it. By comparison, vitamins and minerals are needed in much smaller quantities; thus they are called *micronutrients.* There's a lot of confusion when it comes to understanding the best sources of proteins, but before we get there, let's talk about what a protein is and why the body needs a constant supply of it.

What Is a Protein?

A protein is a compound comprised of carbon, hydrogen, oxygen, and nitrogen arranged as strands of amino acids. These amino acids are the fundamental building blocks of protein. Imagine a Lego tower built from different-colored individual Lego blocks. The entire tower is the protein. It can be short, of medium height, tall, or really tall. Proteins can be all different lengths too. The individual Lego blocks are amino acids. Imagine an enormous box of Lego blocks. You can build many different types of towers of varying colors, sizes, and forms. The same can be said for proteins with one caveat. There are only twenty amino acid building blocks that can be used to build proteins.

You've likely heard the term "amino acid." It's common especially among weight lifters who share notes on the best way to increase their muscle bulk. Sometimes weight lifters will eat amino acid supplements because these are the basic units that the body can use to build proteins. These proteins are important in the repair and building of bigger and stronger muscles.

There are two groups of amino acids, divided according to the body's ability to synthesize them. The first group is comprised of *nonessential* amino acids, so called because the body is able to synthesize them. So if you don't get them in your diet, you don't have to worry because your body will make them. There are eleven nonessential amino acids.

The second group are the *essential* amino acids, so called because the body is *not* able to make them. We must get these amino acids through the foods we eat. There are nine essential amino acids.

Our bodies use the amino acids in our diets to help build proteins that we need to live. This is why it's important to not only have a diet containing adequate amounts of protein, but why the protein we consume must also be of good quality, so that it can be broken down by the body's digestive system and then turned around and used to build new proteins. This is a never-ending process in life as the body is constantly breaking down the proteins in our foods and using them to build new proteins. The body is able to store carbohydrates and fats, but it isn't able to store amino acids. This is why we need to consume a daily diet that contains proteins.

Protein is found throughout our entire body. Muscle, bone, hair, skin, and virtually every other body part or tissue has protein in it. The millions of enzymes in our body that power chemical reactions and the all-important hemoglobin that carries oxygen in our blood are all proteins. There are at least 10,000 proteins that make us who we are.

Not All Protein Is Created Equal

We consume protein from two major sources: animals and plants. Animal proteins are considered to be *high-quality,* or *complete,* proteins because they provide sufficient amounts of the essential amino acids. Animal proteins can be found in such foods as egg, cheese, milk, meat, and fish.

Plant proteins can be found in such sources as grain, corn, nuts, fruits, and vegetables. They are considered to be *lower-quality,* or *incomplete,* proteins because they lack one or more of the essential amino acids or because they lack a proper balance of amino acids. You can, however, combine different plants to get the full spectrum of essential amino acids, but these foods must be consumed at the same time or at least within four hours of each other to get the full benefit.

Vegetarians need to pay attention to the protein sources they're consuming because they don't eat animal proteins.

How Much Protein Do We Need?

Experts haven't unanimously agreed on how much protein we need each day, but they do agree that the majority of Americans are eating more protein than is actually needed. A lot of support in the medical community has been built around the recommendation made by the well-respected Institute of Medicine, which says that adults should get a minimum of 0.8 grams of protein for every kilogram of body weight per day. For example, if you're a 180-pound adult, you should be consuming 65 grams of protein every day. For your own calculations, remember that there are 2.2 pounds per kilogram. So your example might look something like this:

$$\text{Your Weight (155 lbs)} \times \frac{1 \text{ kilogram}}{2.2 \text{ lbs}} \times \frac{0.8 \text{ grams protein}}{1 \text{ kilogram}} = \frac{155 \times 0.8}{2.2} = 56 \text{ grams protein}$$

According to some estimates, adults in the United States consume an average of 15 percent of their calories from protein. For a person who's consuming 2,000 calories a day, that means 300 calories a day in protein. Below is a quick reference guide I've created to give you an idea of how much protein you should be consuming for your weight. Remember, this is just a guide and your specific protein requirement can vary for many reasons, including sickness, level of activity, medications you're taking, etc.

Your Weight (lb)	Your Daily Protein Requirement (g)
130	47
140	51
150	55
160	58

Your Weight (lb)	Your Daily Protein Requirement (g)
170	62
180	65
190	69
200	72
210	76
220	80
230	84
240	87
250	91
260	95
270	98
280	102
290	105
300	109

Where to Get Your Protein

It's important to know not just how much protein is contained in a food, but what the entire protein package looks like. By that I mean what other nutrients and characteristics are present in the food that contains the protein. For example, in a 6-ounce broiled porterhouse steak there are 38 grams of protein—a tremendous amount for such a small volume of food. But while you're getting the amount of protein you want, you're also taking in 44 grams of fat, 16 of which are saturated (the bad kind). By comparison, the same amount of salmon gives you 34 grams of protein, and only 18 grams of fat of which only 4 grams are saturated.[1]

And the salmon provides you with a significant amount of heart-healthy omega-3 fatty acids.

While animal products typically give you the most amount of protein per unit volume of the food you're eating, it's important to be mindful of what else you're getting. A diet high in red meats has repeatedly been shown in studies to increase colon cancer risk.[2] If you're someone who likes red meat, aim for the leanest cuts and choose modest portion sizes (3 to 5 ounces). Eat these red meats occasionally rather than making them a mainstay of your diet. The best-quality animal protein can be found in fish and poultry.

While vegetables don't give you as much bang for your buck when it comes to the amount of protein, they do give you other things that make them worthwhile. The healthy fiber, vitamins, minerals, lower calorie counts, and lower fat counts make vegetables a rewarding source of proteins when you consider the entire package. A cup of lentils, for example, has 18 grams of protein (half what the 6-ounce porterhouse does), but what makes it really healthy protein is that it also contains under 1 gram of fat. By comparison, that porterhouse contained a whopping 44 times more fat.

Following is a simple food chart listing the amounts of protein, calories, and the percentage of the recommended daily value of protein they provide. For example, a 4-ounce serving of yellowfin tuna has only 157.6 calories, but it gives you 34 grams of protein, which is 68 percent of the recommended daily value. The list is in descending order of quality based on the density of protein in the food item.

Food	Serving Size	Calories	Amount of Protein (g)	DV (%)
Cod, baked/broiled	4 oz	119.1	26.03	52.1
Tuna, yellowfin, baked/broiled	4 oz	157.6	33.99	68.0

Food	Serving Size	Calories	Amount of Protein (g)	DV (%)
Shrimp, steamed/ boiled	4 oz	112.3	23.71	47.4
Snapper, baked/ broiled	4 oz	145.2	29.82	59.6
Venison	4 oz	179.2	34.25	68.5
Halibut, baked/ broiled	4 oz	158.8	30.27	60.5
Tamari (soy sauce)	1 Tbsp.	10.8	1.89	3.8
Scallops, baked/ broiled	4 oz	151.7	23.11	46.2
Turkey breast, roasted	4 oz	214.3	32.56	65.1
Chicken breast, roasted	4 oz	223.4	33.79	67.6
Mustard greens, boiled	1 cup	21.0	3.16	6.3
Beef tenderloin, lean, broiled	4 oz	240.4	32.04	64.1
Lamb loin, roasted	4 oz	229.1	30.15	60.3
Calf's liver, braised	4 oz	187.1	24.53	49.1
Spinach, boiled	1 cup	41.4	5.35	10.7
Romaine lettuce	2 cup	15.7	1.81	3.6

continued

Food	Serving Size	Calories	Amount of Protein (g)	DV (%)
Cremini mushrooms, raw	5 oz	31.2	3.54	7.1
Salmon, chinook, baked/broiled	4 oz	261.9	29.14	58.3
Asparagus, boiled	1 cup	43.2	4.66	9.3
Broccoli, steamed	1 cup	43.7	4.66	9.3
Tofu, raw	4 oz	86.2	9.16	18.3
Soybeans, cooked	1 cup	297.6	28.62	57.2
Mozzarella cheese, part-skim, shredded	1 oz	72.1	6.88	13.8
Swiss chard, boiled	1 cup	35.0	3.29	6.6
Tempeh, cooked	4 oz	223.4	20.63	41.3
Yogurt, low-fat	1 cup	155.1	12.86	25.7
Egg, whole, boiled	1 each	68.2	5.54	11.1
Collard greens, boiled	1 cup	49.4	4.01	8.0
Cauliflower, boiled	1 cup	28.5	2.28	4.6
Lentils, cooked	1 cup	229.7	17.86	35.7

Food	Serving Size	Calories	Amount of Protein (g)	DV (%)
Split peas, cooked	1 cup	231.3	16.35	32.7
Kidney beans, cooked	1 cup	224.8	15.35	30.7
Kale, boiled	1 cup	36.4	2.47	4.9
Lima beans, cooked	1 cup	216.2	14.66	29.3
Black beans, cooked	1 cup	227.0	15.24	30.5
Cow's milk, 2%	1 cup	121.2	8.13	16.3
Brussel sprouts, boiled	1 cup	60.8	3.98	8.0
Green peas, boiled	1 cup	134.4	8.58	17.2
Navy beans, cooked	1 cup	258.4	15.83	31.7
Pinto beans, cooked	1 cup	234.3	14.04	28.1
Miso	1 oz	70.8	4.06	8.1
Shiitake mushrooms, raw	8 oz	87.2	4.98	10.0
Turnip greens, cooked	1 cup	28.8	1.64	3.3
Garbanzo beans (chickpeas), cooked	1 cup	269.0	14.53	29.1

continued

Food	Serving Size	Calories	Amount of Protein (g)	DV (%)
Green beans, boiled	1 cup	43.8	2.36	4.7
Mustard seeds	2 tsp	35.0	1.88	3.8
Goat's milk	1 cup	167.9	8.69	17.4
Cabbage, shredded, boiled	1 cup	33.0	1.53	3.1
Summer squash, cooked, slices	1 cup	36.0	1.64	3.3
Peanuts, raw	0.25 cup	207.0	9.42	18.8
Pumpkin seeds, raw	0.25 cup	186.7	8.47	16.9
Rye, whole grain, uncooked	0.33 cup	188.7	8.31	16.6
Spelt grains, cooked	4 oz	144.0	6.24	12.5
Garlic	1 oz	42.2	1.80	3.6
Oats, whole grain, cooked	1 cup	147.4	6.08	12.2
Tomato, ripe	1 cup	37.8	1.53	3.1

Source: The World's Healthiest Foods

So many foods contain protein that it's not always easy to know which sources give you the biggest protein bang for your buck. For various reasons, millions of people are looking to beef up their protein intake—whether it's weight lifters trying to bulk up or those who are trying to lose weight. The following are five tables that give you the best sources of protein for meats; poultry; seafood; dairy; and vegetables, grains, beans, and legumes. (Note, the dairy table also provides information on fat.) The protein content is calculated for 100 grams or 3.5 ounces of that particular food. For fish and meat, this is a portion size roughly three quarter the size of a deck of cards.

Meat Protein Source (100 g)	Amount of Protein (g)
Pork bacon	37.0
Buffalo (bison) steak, top round	29.5
Beef, top sirloin, steak	29.5
Beef, flank steak	27.6
Beef, rib-eye	27.3
Beef, skirt steak	26.7
Lamb, loin chops	26.6
Pork, tenderloin	26.0
Beef, ground, 95% lean meat	25.2
Beef, tenderloin	23.9
Duck, without skin	23.5
Beef, prime rib	22.9
Pork, sausage, fresh	19.4
Duck, with skin	19.0
Beef, sausage, fresh	18.2

Poultry Protein Source (100 g)	Amount of Protein (g)
Chicken breast, without skin, grilled or roasted	31.0
Chicken breast, with skin, grilled or roasted	29.8
Turkey bacon	29.6
Turkey breast, without skin	29.3
Turkey breast with skin	28.7
Venison ground, cooked	26.5
Turkey, ground 93% lean	25.9
Chicken breast, ground, lean	23.3
Chicken breast, cold cut	19.9

Seafood Protein Source (100 g)	Amount of Protein (g)
Tuna, Yellow fin (tuna steak)	29.5
Tuna, light: canned in oil, drained solids	29.1
Tuna, light: canned in water, drained solids	25.5
Salmon, Atlantic, wild, cooked, dry heat	25.4
Sardines: canned in oil, drained solids with bone	24.6
Mackerel, Atlantic, cooked, dry heat	23.9
Sea bass, cooked, dry heat	23.6
Mackerel, jack, canned, drained solids	23.2
Cod, Atlantic, cooked, dry heat	22.8
Halibut, Atlantic and Pacific, cooked, dry heat	22.5
Herring, Pacific, cooked, dry heat	21.0
Catfish, wild, cooked, dry heat	18.5

Seafood Protein Source (100 g)	Amount of Protein (g)
Perch, cooked, dry heat	18.5
Squid, mixed species, cooked, fried	17.9

Dairy Sources of Protein and Fat

Milk and Dairy Products	Serving Size	Total Calories	Grams Protein	Grams Fat
Buttermilk (low-fat, with active cultures)	1 cup	98	8	2
Cheddar cheese (low-fat)	1 oz / 1 slice	48	7	2
Cottage cheese (2% low-fat)	½ cup	97	13	3
Cottage cheese (non-fat)	½ cup	81	12	0
Cream cheese (low-fat)	1 Tbsp.	30	1	2
Cream cheese (non-fat)	1 Tbsp.	15	2	0
Milk (whole)	1 cup	146	8	8
Milk (1% fat)	1 cup	102	8	2
Milk (skim/ nonfat)	1 cup	86	8	0
Monterey Jack	1 oz / 1 slice	88	8	6

continued

Milk and Dairy Products	Serving Size	Total Calories	Grams Protein	Grams Fat
Mozzarella (part skim milk)	1 oz	71	7	4
Provolone (reduced fat)	1 oz / 1 slice	77	7	5
Ricotta (part skim milk)	1/2 cup	171	14	10
Swiss cheese	1 oz / 1 slice	50	8	1
*Yogurt (low-fat, added fruit)	1 cup	243	10	3
Yogurt, Greek	1/2 cup	70	14	0
*Vanilla ice cream	1/2 cup	137	2	7

Reference: NutritionData.com

*Yogurt and ice cream brands vary greatly in the amount of calories in proportion to the amount of protein. Be sure to read and compare labels, even if they say low-fat, since many of these products have added sugars and/or fruit.

Vegetables/Grains/Beans/Legumes (100 g)	Amount of Protein (g)
Lentils	9.0
Pinto beans	9.0
Black beans, boiled	8.9
Chickpeas (garbanzo beans), boiled	8.9
Kidney beans	8.7
Lima beans	7.8

Vegetables/Grains/Beans/Legumes (100 g)	Amount of Protein (g)
Navy beans, canned	7.5
Navy beans, boiled	7.1
Kidney beans, canned	5.2
Baked beans, canned	5.2
Chickpeas (garbanzo beans), canned	5.0
Lima beans, canned	4.9
Pinto beans, canned	4.9
Baked potatoes, white	4.3
Wild rice	4.0
Lentil soup with ham, ready to serve	3.7
Oatmeal, instant, prepared with water	3.6
White rice	2.4
Oatmeal, old-fashioned	2.4
Brown rice	2.3
Baked sweet potato	2.0

Not Enough Protein

Low protein intake is typically not a problem in the industrialized Western Hemisphere; we get *more* than enough protein in our diets. Americans consume an average of 15 percent of their daily calories from this important macronutrient, putting us safely within the 10 to 35 percent range currently recommended by the U.S. Department of Agriculture. In the U.S. and other developed countries, getting enough protein in the diet is quite easy. According to the Harvard School of Public Health, cereal with milk for breakfast, a peanut butter and jelly sandwich for lunch, and a piece of fish with a side of beans for dinner adds up to about 70 grams of protein, which is typically more than enough for the average adult. However, some people with poor or altered diets are not consuming the proper level of protein.

Protein plays a critical role in muscle repair and development. A sustained low protein intake could lead to a loss of muscle. According to a study published in the *American Journal of Clinical Nutrition* (May 2007), inadequate protein intake can lead to impaired muscle function and reduced muscle strength, both difficult conditions since they can lead to weight loss and loss of energy. Poor protein intake can also mean it takes longer for muscles to recover from injury, whether it's the natural injury experienced with strength training or accidental "injury from something like a strain or pull."

Hair growth can also suffer as a result of inadequate protein intake. While it's not common in the United States, those suffering from severe protein deficiency can experience growth failure, decreased immunity, and weakening of the heart and respiratory system. When the protein deficiency isn't corrected, this condition can lead to death.

Too Much Protein

While there are many benefits to having protein in our diets, in recent years there has been an obsession with protein-rich diets when it comes to weight loss and enhancing athletic performance. Many erroneously believe that if eating a moderate amount of protein is good, then eating even more means they can achieve even better results. This is not only false, it can be dangerous.

Diets high in protein typically have not proven to be a serious hazard for people who are generally in good health. This is not the case, however, for someone suffering from kidney or liver disease. When proteins are broken down into amino acids and the number of amino acids are in excess of the number the body can use, what remains is supposed to be excreted by the kidneys and liver. If someone's kidney and/or liver isn't functioning correctly, this extra protein load can overwhelm them. The nitrogen wastes start to accumulate in both the liver and kidneys and cause problems. Experts also believe that these high-protein diets may increase the risk of kidney stones and osteoporosis.

Another concern about high-protein diets is the source of the protein. Many people try to consume the extra protein by eating animal products such as red processed meats. These meats can have extremely high levels of saturated fat, and many studies have shown that prolonged consumption of foods rich in animal fat can increase a person's risk for coronary heart disease, diabetes, stroke, and several types of cancer.

Soy Protein

The soybean is a powerful little package that contains all three of the macronutrients (carbohydrates, fats, and protein) as well as vitamins and minerals. Calcium, folic acid, and iron—three critical nutrients for many of our life processes—are also found in this health-filled bean. Soybeans are well distinguished in that they're the only common plant food that contains complete protein, which means soy provides all of the essential amino acids needed for human health. A half cup of cooked mature soybeans delivers an impressive 14.3 grams of protein, while half a cup of green baby soybeans (edamame) delivers 11.1 grams.

Soy is extremely popular with people who are looking for healthy alternatives, whether it is consumed as milk, beans, or nuts. Over the last fifteen years soy really came into fashion: every week there seemed to be a new health claim about the benefits of soy consumption. The most notable and widespread claim has been that a diet containing 25 grams of soy protein—which is also low in saturated fat and cholesterol—may reduce the risk of heart disease. In 1999, the FDA stepped into the arena in an attempt to bring some calm and stability to the many claims. The FDA gave manufacturers of foods high in soy protein permission to make claims that they *may* help lower heart disease. However, there were specific criteria that had to be met. Each serving of the particular food must contain:

    6.25 grams of soy protein
    less than 3 grams of fat
    less than 1 gram of saturated fat
    less than 20 milligrams cholesterol
    less than 480 milligrams sodium for individual foods, less than
        720 milligrams sodium for main dish, and less than 960 milligrams
        sodium for complete meal

There has been significant controversy about some of the other soy health claims. Many people have voiced strong opinions that soy has helped with the hot flashes of menopause, reduced the risk of breast cancer, and improved memory and cognitive ability. At best, the studies have been contradictory and so there hasn't been consensus as to whether high soy consumption really can deliver all that many believe and hope it can. But even if soy doesn't live up to all of the hype, the majority of experts do agree that soy is a great addition to our diets and a significantly better alternative to some of the typical fare we consume that provides little in the way of nutritional value and lots in the way of calories and fats.

Tips for Adding Protein to Your Diet

◆ Add protein-rich vegetables to your salads and include them more often as side dishes in your meals. Some of these vegetables include: green peas, broccoli, cauliflower, asparagus, watercress, brussels sprouts, and spinach. Steam them in the microwave or add them to your salad.

◆ Add meat, but make sure to choose the leanest of cuts since meat can contain large amounts of saturated fats. Poultry is wonderful, but eat it without the skin. Simply add grilled chicken strips to your salad or meat to your soup.

◆ Add whole grains. Along with many other healthy nutrients, whole grains contain respectable levels of protein. Increase your intake of quinoa, brown rice, whole wheat, oat bran, and other whole grains (see chapter 3). You can make buckwheat pancakes instead of pancakes from white flour. Add oat bran to those homemade muffins. Quinoa is a great thickener that can be added to your soups and stews.

◆ Add seafood. These oceangoing critters are a great source of heart-healthy nutrients as well as protein. Scallops, fresh tuna, salmon, clams, halibut, and cod are just some of the many seafood items that can make a difference. Add shrimp to your pasta or salad, include tuna in your whole wheat pita sandwich, or eat some steamed clams as an appetizer in a restaurant.

◆ Add soy. Tofu is very popular and flexible. It has virtually no taste, so it can absorb the flavors of the foods that it's mixed with. Tofu can be easily added to your soups or stir-fry. Snack on delicious edamame (baby soy beans), very lightly salted. Instead of a glass of regular milk, try a glass of soy milk.

◆ Try an egg. While they are heavy in cholesterol, eggs offer a broad spectrum of nutrients, particularly vitamin B, vitamin A, vitamin D, vitamin E, and vitamin K. One large egg has almost 6 grams of protein. If you want to avoid the cholesterol, then try eating egg whites.

continued

You can make egg white omelettes with peppers and onions, getting lots of protein and fewer calories and fats.

◆ Add beans and (fresh or canned) legumes. Black beans, kidney beans, soybeans, lentils, chickpeas, pinto beans, and lima beans are a great source of protein. Dip your veggies in chickpea hummus, oven roast chickpeas for a snack, microwave a cup of black bean soup and mix in diced chicken.

◆ Don't forget the dairy. Milk, cheese, yogurt, and cottage cheese can boost your protein. Choose low fat or fat free. It won't change the amount of protein, but will make it a healthier package.

EAT Plan

◆ Be *proactive* about your *protein*. First, get an idea of how much you should be consuming daily by using the quick-reference guide in the beginning of the chapter. Try to divide your day's protein between your meals and snacks, making sure not to consume more than a third of your requirement at one sitting.

◆ Eat good protein packages. Remember, it's not just the protein, but the other nutrients and calories that come along with the food that contains the protein. Consume at least half of your daily protein requirement from the best packages: vegetables, grains, beans, and legumes.

◆ Be mindful of the calories in dairy products. Just switching from regular to a reduced-fat product can save calories.

◆ Skin your meat protein and keep it out of the fryer. Naked chicken and turkey means you will eat fewer calories naturally and keep the protein bonds of the meat intact (the heat of frying can denature the protein bonds).

Spicetopia

Five of the Tastiest and Healthiest Spices in the World

- ✦ Gifts from a Green Earth
- ✦ Spicing Up Your Health
- ✦ Salt Galore—a Crisis
- ✦ Flavorful Cooking Tips

Spices are truly the magical little wonders of good eating. I was not raised on a lot of spices, since my grandfather—who lived with us—preferred his foods so bland they were practically tasteless. But as I grew older and began sampling foods that were prepared outside of our home, I began to discover the amazing powers of spices and how they could transform the most basic of foods—say a grilled chicken breast—and make them taste as if prepared for a king's feast.

One of the greatest advantages of spices is that they have virtually no calories. You can add them to your soups, meats, vegetables, and fish and come away with a dish that has completely changed in terms of taste, but has remained unchanged when it comes to calorie count. If you think "healthy" food isn't tasty, welcome to the wonderful world of spices.

Spices even give us something beyond the kick in taste and no calories. These plant-derived compounds, whose use dates back thousands of years, can also deliver a dose of health benefits. Historically, culinary herbs and spices were used as both medicines and food preservatives. Historians have noted that ancient Egyptians as far back as 1555 BC classified coriander, fennel, juniper, cumin, garlic, and thyme as health-promoting spices. It's been documented that laborers who constructed the Great Pyramid of Cheops ate onion and garlic in an effort to promote health. The following pages highlight spices that will not only make your food more agreeable to your palate, but will help your body fight disease. Because these spices can be quite potent in their medical properties, it's always advised that you consult with your physician and discuss if you use them in very high quantities or as supplements. They can have interactions with medications you're taking and impact the course and outcome of many medical conditions.

Thrill of Eating

Good eating is one of life's greatest pleasures. Food not only answers our physiological needs as human beings, but it can be a great way to share quality time with our loved ones. One of the worst things we can do is lose our zest and curiosity about food. Focusing on calories and health implications is important, but too much focus can ruin our gastronomic experiences. Unfortunately, too many people think healthy eating has to be boring, that healthy food actually has to taste bad. Instead, they beg you to bring on the fried foods and meats slathered in barbecue sauce. In their minds, the best-tasting food is the food that's the least healthy.

How we mix our foods, cook our foods, and the spices we add to them can add up to a terrific eating experience. Often we are too impatient or too set in our ways to try new cuisines and flavors. We are too reluctant to experiment in our own kitchens with recipes that prepare traditional dishes in a new way. Those who have found the balance between eating healthfully and eating tastefully will tell you how lucky they are to have the best of both worlds. But it's really not about luck. You can make a conscious decision to seek out ways to enrich your foods with taste and still benefit from the nourishment that healthy food provides. Spices can be the key to accomplishing this.

Garlic

Garlic is one of the most studied, most widely used plants in the history of civilization, dating back some 5,000 to 6,000 years. It was native to Central Asia and spread rapidly eastward throughout China, southward to India, and westward to the Mediterranean. From the very beginning, garlic has been used both as a food and as a medicinal product. It was of great importance to the Egyptians, who believed it created strength and stamina; they fed it to the slaves who built the pyramids. The ancient Indians thought garlic was an aphrodisiac. The ancient Greeks and Romans used it to repel scorpions, treat bladder infections, and cure leprosy and asthma. Even as recent as World War II, garlic was used as an antiseptic to disinfect open wounds and prevent the development of gangrene.

Ironically, garlic was not well received in America for decades. It was largely believed to be an ethnic ingredient and not a flavor that was appealing to a mainstream palate. But by the early 1940s, with the more widespread use of the herb and the wider acceptance of ethnic cuisines, garlic was fully embraced by Americans. In fact, it's estimated that Americans consume more than 250 million pounds of garlic annually.

Garlic has been lovingly nicknamed "The Stinking Rose," but the truth is that it's really a member of the lily family, which also includes onions, shallots, chives, and leeks. It is considered to be a root crop, because the bulb grows underground. This bulb, or head, is comprised of several pungent bulblets called cloves. There are more than 300 varieties of garlic grown worldwide; approximately 90 percent of the garlic grown in the United States is grown in California. Its distinctively pungent taste and smell are due to a chemical reaction that occurs when the garlic cells are ruptured by either cutting or pressing. This flavor is most intense immediately after cutting, chopping, or pressing. The reaction that produces this flavor occurs in the raw state and can't happen after the garlic has been cooked. This is why roasted garlic is sweet rather than pungent.

There is lots of folklore about the therapeutic benefits of garlic, and there are also plenty of valid medical claims. Garlic is full of vitamins—including A, B, and C—as well as a broad spectrum of other nutrients and minerals—such as iodine, calcium, zinc, magnesium, folate, potassium, protein, and selenium.

Much of the modern research on garlic has focused on garlic's ability to lower cholesterol and blood pressure as well as protect against strokes and heart disease. When the *Journal of the Royal College of Physicians* reviewed data on cholesterol, it found that after just four weeks there was a 12 percent reduction in cholesterol levels in the participant groups that took garlic supplements.[1] A 2008 study found that 600 milligrams of daily garlic supplementation significantly decreases LDL ("bad") cholesterol and increases HDL "good" cholesterol within twelve weeks of treatment.[2]

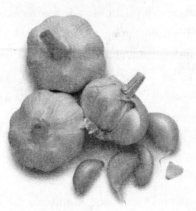

Abnormal blood clots—a dangerous medical situation that can lead to dire consequences—were put to the test against the power of garlic. Research has found that those who regularly take garlic have longer blood clotting times, which means a lowered risk of developing the dangerous blood clots that can lead to heart attacks, strokes, and lung problems. A review of clinical trials published in the *Journal of Hypertension* showed that taking garlic tablets cut the participants' blood pressure by between 1 and 5 percent. From this information, the researchers concluded that taking garlic supplements could reduce the incidence of heart disease by 20 to 25 percent and stroke by 30 to 40 percent.

Garlic has also been found to help fight against bacteria, viruses, yeast, and stomach cancer.

How you prepare or cook garlic can make a big difference in its taste. To get the biggest bang for your buck, finely mince or press the garlic to release maximum flavor. One rule of thumb is the smaller you cut it, the stronger the flavor. The more finely you chop and/or press it, the more surface area of the clove you expose to the air, causing more of the chemical reaction that produces garlic's pungent aroma and flavor. When garlic cloves are not cut up, but instead cooked or baked whole, the flavor calms into a sweet, almost nutty flavor that barely resembles its pungency when raw. Surprisingly, for a plant that can fill a room with its distinctive aroma, garlic cloves that are cooked, whole, or un-pierced barely have any aroma at all.

Ginger

Ginger has a tremendously long history, dating back some 5,000 years to southeastern Asia where it was used both in food and in medicine. According to Michael Castleman in *The Healing Herbs,* the ancient Greeks wrapped ginger inside their bread and ate it as an after-dinner digestive to prevent nausea after a huge feast. Some believe this practice eventually led to the invention of gingerbread. For many centuries Chinese sailors have taken ginger to avoid seasickness. The English created ginger beer to soothe the stomach, and in the 1800s, a medical reform sect called the Eclectics used ginger powder and ginger tea to treat several digestive problems including gas, nausea, indigestion, and infant diarrhea. (See page 107 for a ginger tea recipe.)

Successfully growing ginger requires a hot, moist climate with plenty of sunshine and rain, which explains why it's primarily cultivated in tropical regions. The majority of ginger is currently grown in China, India, Jamaica, and Hawaii. While most people are familiar with the term "gingerroot" as a major source for food and supplements, the truth is that we eat not the actual root but rather the plant's underground stem, the rhizome. Ginger is available in seven major forms—fresh, pickled (called *gari* or *beni shoga* in Japan and often eaten with sushi), preserved (an Asian specialty that's preserved in a sugar-salt mixture), crystallized or candied (cooked in a sugar syrup), juice, dried, ground or powdered (the most popular form of the spice).

Ginger contains several chemical components that include starch, protein, lipids, protease (enzyme), volatile oils, pungent principles, and vitamins A and B3 (nicacin). The special compounds called pungent principles are believed to be the most medicinally potent as they can influence blood flow and inflammation. These compounds also give ginger its sharp and highly recognizable aroma.[3]

The medicinal claims for ginger are widespread and in some cases nothing but rich folklore. Ginger has been used as an anti-inflammatory

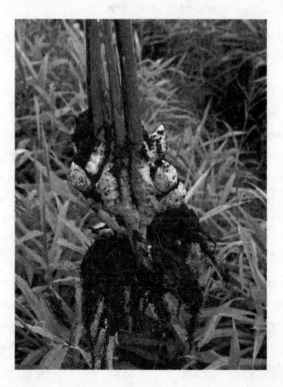

to reduce pain and swelling, an aid to digestion, and a treatment for loss of appetite. Over the last couple of decades scientists have sought to find some definitive answers about what we can expect from this ubiquitous plant, and have put ginger under rigorous research on its effectiveness and safety. Unfortunately, a lot of the studies are either inconclusive or contradictory. But the National Center for Complementary and Alternative Medicine has this to say about the benefits of ginger:

- Studies suggest that the short-term use of ginger can safely relieve pregnancy-related nausea and vomiting.
- Studies are mixed on whether ginger is effective for nausea caused by motion, chemotherapy, or surgery.
- It is unclear whether ginger is effective for treating rheumatoid arthritis, osteoarthritis, or joint and muscle pain.

Could the ancients all be wrong? The point is well taken that just because scientific studies have yet to conclusively determine the medicinal properties of ginger, it certainly doesn't mean they don't exist. While the way we currently study and research compounds may not have been around hundreds and thousands of years ago, it would be arrogant and small-minded at best to presume that the wisdom of those who've predated us was false simply because they didn't have the high-powered laboratories and stringent scientific protocols we have today.

Fresh ginger has a tangy freshness, warmth, mellow sweetness, and a light spiciness. It can be used in combination with other spices and flavors or used simply as a dominant flavor. It is a great complement to meat, poultry, and fish dishes. To get the full brunt of the raw ginger, cut, chop, mince, or grate it, then add it to the dish just before serving. Just like garlic, fresh ginger mellows with cooking, and turns bitter if you burn it. Fresh ginger can be found year-round in the produce section of most supermarkets. Look for smooth skin with a fresh, spicy fragrance. Length is a sign of maturity. Be careful to avoid those with wrinkled flesh, because this is a sign the ginger is past its prime. The ground or powdered form of ginger has a much different flavor from the other forms and is typically used to make sweet desserts. Fresh ginger and ground ginger are very different and typically not interchangeable, so if a recipe calls for one, don't assume you can simply substitute it with the other.

Quick and Easy Ginger Tea Recipe

INGREDIENTS

4 to 6 thin slices raw ginger (or $3/4$ teaspoon ground ginger)
2 cups water
1–2 tablespoons honey
Fresh lime juice from $1/2$ lime

Cut the ginger slices so that they are thin and have the most amount of surface area exposed. Pour the water in a saucepan, then add the ginger slices. Bring the water to boil and continue boiling for 8 to 10 minutes. Then remove the saucepan from heat and strain the tea. Add honey and lime juice if desired.

Cinnamon

Whenever I think of cinnamon, my mind conjures up images of the ground reddish brown spice being added to French toast batter. A favorite spice of mine since childhood, I had not the slightest inkling that cinnamon also carries with it an assortment of health benefits.

Cinnamon is an aromatic spice that's available in two major forms—stick and ground powder. The spice is harvested from the inner bark of the cinnamon tree, which is stripped off and allowed to dry in the sun. As the bark is drying, it rolls up into a quill, which we know as a cinnamon stick. These sticks can also be ground down into a powder. That's what my mother put in our French toast batter.

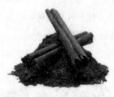

Cinnamon, like many other popular spices, dates back thousands of years to southern Asia where the Chinese used it to treat fever, diarrhea, and menstrual problems. The ancient Ayurvedic healers in India used it similarly, and the Egyptians added it to their embalming mixtures. When the Greeks and Romans adopted it as a spice, perfume, and treatment for indigestion, it became one of the world's most popular and heavily sought-after commodities. In America in the mid-nineteenth century, the Eclectic physicians (branch of physicians who used botanical remedies along with other alternative therapies) used it regularly to treat nausea, vomiting, diarrhea, uterine problems, infant colic, flatulence, and stomach cramps.

Cinnamon contains several nutrients including manganese, dietary fiber, iron, and calcium. But it also contains a group of essential oils that are believed to be responsible for its healing powers. While many studies have looked at the medicinal properties of cinnamon, scientists have yet to voice a unanimous opinion on what we might expect therapeutically from regular use of cinnamon. There is, however, a growing body of evidence that is suggestive of several of cinnamon's health benefits. These include:

- Thinning the blood to reduce abnormal clotting
- Stopping growth of bacteria and fungi
- Helping to stabilize and in some cases lower blood sugar levels
- Lowering cholesterol and triglyceride levels in diabetics

Both the ground and stick forms of cinnamon are equally healthy, but cinnamon sticks have a longer shelf life.

Turmeric

This golden-colored, earthy, bitter spice with a mild fragrance slightly reminiscent of orange and ginger is considered one of the most versatile spices available. Used for over 4,000 years to treat a variety of ailments in Chinese and Ayurvedic medicine, turmeric is widely grown throughout India, as well as other parts of Asia and Africa. It's been nicknamed "Indian saffron" because of its deep yellow-orange color and immense popularity in a country where it was most likely first used as a dye and now is primarily used as a major ingredient in curry.

Turmeric comes from the underground stem of the *Curcuma longa* plant, which is in the ginger family. While it's commonly referred to as a root, that is not anatomically correct. It's actually the stem, or rhizome, of the plant that grows underground *above* the root. Turmeric "root" has a tough brown skin and a deep orange flesh. Similar to ginger, the chopped or powdered root has a tart taste, but turmeric's flavor is mustier and contains peppery undertones. Turmeric can be purchased in both "root" and powder form, though the powder form is far more popular. Hardcore foodies who want fresh turmeric powder are willing to put in a little extra labor to find it, peel it, boil it, dry it, then grind it to a fine consistency.

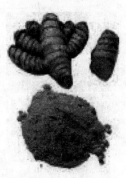

Some of the nutrients found in turmeric include manganese, iron, vitamin B_6, dietary fiber, and potassium. Long used for its anti-inflammatory properties, the active ingredient in turmeric is believed to be curcumin, which is also responsible for turmeric's yellow coloring. Western science has not yet fully investigated all the health claims associated with turmeric, but there is a growing belief that this ancient spice may have promise in fighting infections and some cancers as well as reducing inflammation and treating digestive problems. Research suggests that turmeric could be helpful in treating the following conditions:

- Rheumatoid arthritis/osteoarthritis
- Inflammatory bowel disease
- Cancer (prostate, breast, skin, and colon among others)
- Stomach ulcers

- Indigestion or dyspepsia
- Heart disease (atherosclerosis)
- Diabetes
- Bacterial and viral infections
- Alzheimer's disease

Turmeric is a cook's dream spice because of its flexibility. It improves any kind of poultry or seafood by giving it a warm color and accentuating the natural flavor of the dish. Turmeric is also a great ingredient to be added to rice, lentils, vegetables, salads, soups, and stews. Many creative chefs use it for everything from fried chicken seasoning to pumping up the mayonnaise in potato salad. Use turmeric sparingly since it has such a strong taste that gets stronger the longer you cook it. A little goes a long way. One little warning: turmeric is a powerful dye so be careful not to get it on your clothes.

Cayenne Pepper

Two words: "hot" and "spicy"! These are the key characteristics of this powerful spice that was originally grown in Central and South America in pre-Columbian times before spreading to Europe thanks to the explorations of Christopher Columbus. Currently grown in tropical regions around the world, it's used by many countries for its powerful medical properties.

Cayenne pepper is a member of the *Capsicum* genus that includes such items as Tabasco peppers, Mexican chili peppers, bell peppers, pimentos, paprikas, and African bird peppers. While many might think a famous rock band—Red Hot Chili Peppers—might have invented the name, the true credit goes to the ancient Aztecs who called cayenne pepper chili. This plant, which grows to a height of two to six feet, typically produces long, tapering red peppers (green if picked before ripening). While the peppers themselves can be chopped and added to foods, most people use powdered cayenne, which is the result of grinding the dried flesh and seeds of the red pepper. Typically, the redder the pepper, the hotter it is, except for a few exceptions such as the yellow Scotch bonnet pepper.

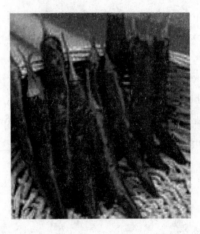

Cayenne peppers are full of nutrients, including vitamins A, B_6, C, and K; manganese; and dietary fiber. But the heat is caused by the high concentration of a compound called capsaicin, one that has been well-studied in medical literature. The more capsaicin the pepper contains, the hotter it is. The hottest varieties are habañero, Scotch bonnet, and cayenne peppers. The famous jalapeños fall in the next hottest group.

Beyond providing the heat, capsaicin is largely responsible for cayenne pepper's well-documented medical properties. It is widely used as a pain reliever, because it reduces the amount of substance P, a chemical that sends pain signals to the brain. When there's less of substance P, our awareness of pain diminishes because the pain signal can't reach the brain. Capsaicin is a major ingredient in some over-the-counter creams used to treat everything from the pain of shingles to rheumatic and arthritic pains, cluster headaches, diabetic foot pain, and fibromyalgia.

Cayenne has also been reported to be an effective remedy for relieving congestion and coughs because it thins the mucus and thus improves the flow of bodily fluids. Other potential benefits include: aiding digestion, relieving constipation, lowering cholesterol levels, lowering the risk of blood clots, lowering blood pressure, fighting inflammation, and boosting the immune system.

Cooking with cayenne pepper can be lots of fun, but you must know what you're doing. When it comes to this sizzling spice, a little truly goes a long way. You can add a pinch to soups or meats, salad dressings and sauces. Using the entire pepper will give you the hottest flavor. If you want to cool it down, simply remove and discard the seeds and/or veins inside of the pepper. When using cayenne while cooking, add it gradually to avoid using too much. Add a pinch, stir, cook for several minutes, then taste to see if it's where you want the flavor to be. One tip to reduce the burn from this pepper if you do overdo it: hold milk or yogurt in your mouth.

Cut the Salt (the Honorary Spice)

America is drowning in salt—literally. Our favorite of all spices, it's easy to overdo. A recent report by the CDC found that nine out of ten Americans eat too much salt, with most getting more than twice the recommended amount. When I first heard about these findings, I wasn't surprised. How many times have you been at the dinner table when a relative hasn't just sprinkled salt on their food, but literally poured it on? But when I read the details of the report, I really was surprised. Researchers estimate that 77 percent of the dietary sodium we consume comes from processed and restaurant foods. The biggest culprit isn't Uncle Robert's liberal shaking as he adds a layer of tiny white salt crystals, but rather the food we purchase that is already drenched in sodium.

The 2005 dietary guidelines for Americans recommended we eat no more than 2,300 milligrams of sodium per day, which is about one teaspoon. The guidelines that were recently proposed for 2010 lowered that recommendation to 1,500 milligrams, especially for those considered to be part of the high-risk groups (people with high blood pressure, middle-aged and older adults, and African-Americans), which amounts to 145.5 million people. What's so alarming is that most Americans consume 3,466 milligrams of sodium per day, dramatically more than what's needed and considered healthy.

There's simply so much salt in our food chain that it's becoming increasingly difficult to stay within the recommended limits. Reducing the amount of salt we add at the table will make a difference, but more will need to be done on the part of manufacturers of processed foods. The Institute of Medicine has called on the FDA to start regulating how much salt is added to foods, hoping this will help Americans cut back on their salt intake. The FDA has yet to make a decision on this mandate, and there could be a long, hard-fought battle from both sides of the table. But this doesn't mean consumers can't practice better habits right now by reading the ingredient label for the sodium content of foods and being more conservative when they tip the salt shaker. Much of the excess sodium in our diets comes from foods like pizza, cookies, meats, and canned products. In fact, grain-based foods, meat, chicken, and fish account for nearly two thirds of our daily salt intake. Health experts are sounding the alarm because it's well documented that eating too much salt can raise blood pressure, which can lead to a domino-effect of negative health consequences, including kidney failure, strokes, and heart disease.

There's no denying that salt can add tremendous flavor to foods. But exercising moderation and making smart choices can allow us to continue to enjoy our favorite spice without putting ourselves at risk for illness.

Tips for Adding Spices to Your Diet

✦ Measure your spices and herbs in a measuring cup or spoon, then add them to food as it's cooking. Avoid sprinkling spices and herbs directly from their bottles since repeated exposure to heat and moisture can accelerate flavor loss and result in caking.

✦ Choose ground spices over whole spices—they release their flavor more quickly. If cooking dishes that take more time, consider whole spices because they release their flavor more slowly.

✦ It's best to add crushed, powdered, or ground spices during the last 15 minutes of cooking since they release their flavors faster than whole spices.

✦ To get the most flavor, dried whole herbs and spices should be replaced every year. Ground/powdered spices should be replaced every six months.

✦ Toast whole spices over high heat in a dry, heavy pan before grinding them into a powder. This will help release more flavor from the spice.

continued

◆ Rub your meat. Brush both sides of your steak or pork chop with olive oil, then apply a mixture of salt, ground black pepper, thyme, garlic powder, onion powder, and whatever other spice you like. Use your fingers or fork to push the rub into the meat. Let the meat sit and marinate for at least 15 minutes before cooking.

◆ Warm a powdered spice or herb in a little bit of olive oil before adding it to the food you're cooking. This will best bring out the flavor of the spice when adding it to your food.

EAT Plan

◆ Every two weeks add a new spice to your cooking/eating. Pay particular attention to the blander foods such as rice, pasta dishes, and skinless chicken. Mix up the spices to create variety.

◆ A little bit of spice goes a long way. Use spices sparingly so that you don't overpower the food. Typically a ½ teaspoon of most spices is sufficient for a dish that's serving four people. Experiment with the quantity until you're satisfied.

◆ Because ground spices and herbs release their flavors quite readily, when preparing long-cooking dishes, add them near the end of the cooking time so that the flavor doesn't "cook off or dissipate." For uncooked foods such as salads, add the spices and herbs to the dressing several hours before eating to allow the flavors to develop and blend.

7
Size Matters

- ✦ Secret Calories You Don't Know About
- ✦ Size Your Servings Made Simple
- ✦ Cut Portions, Cut Your Weight
- ✦ Fast Food Under 500 Calories

*B*ig is not always better—even in Texas. The world is currently battling an obesity epidemic that's showing no signs of letting up. Many industrialized nations find their waistlines expanding, their scales tipping, and their risks for various medical conditions jumping to levels never seen before. To make matters worse, the United States is disgracefully leading the pack. The Organisation for Economic Cooperation and Development (OECD) took a look at the major industrialized nations around the world and compared their rates of obesity and overweight.[1] It found the U.S. at the top of the list with 64.5 percent of its population over weight, followed by Mexico at 62.3 percent, the

United Kingdom at 61 percent, and Australia at 58.4 percent. The two nations with the lowest percentages? Japan at 25.8 percent and Korea at 30.6 percent.

While it has become almost a sport in the last ten years to blame carbohydrates for our weight struggles, the truth is that physical inactivity and outrageous portion sizes are really the co-stars. They are the driving forces behind these exploding obesity rates. Size really does matter, especially when it comes to what you're putting on your plate and then into your mouth.

Portions Gone Wild

Over the last twenty years, the amount of food that we sit down and consume at one meal has literally spiraled out of control. Thanks to all-you-can-eat buffets, buy-one-get-one-free deals, and the supersizing of everything from soft drinks to hot dogs, we are packing in calories in record numbers. Take a look at the change in our daily calorie intake over a thirty-year period.

Average Calorie Intake per Day

	1971	2000	Change
Women	1,542	1,877	Up 22%
Men	2,450	2,618	Up 7%

Source: "Trends in Intake of Energy and Macronutrients—United States 1971-2000," Center for Disease Control and Prevention, *MMWR Weekly*, February 6, 2004.

And this chart is only for information we have up to the year 2000. The more current numbers are still being compiled, but it's certain they are going to be even worse. Some estimates are putting the average daily intake of calories for everyone at over 3,000. Say all you want about good carbs and bad carbs, but the simple truth is that we have been and are continuing to literally eat our way into obesity and its related medical complications such as type 2 diabetes, heart disease, stroke, high blood pressure, and some forms of cancer.

Without thinking much about the consequences to our health or cooks, we have adopted a philosophy of "more is better." During the early days of "supersizing," manufacturers and consumers were tickled pink. The manufacturers and food retailers were excited because they had figured out a way to increase their profits by increasing the portions they served or making portions unlimited (the all-you-can-eat buffets) for higher prices to consumers who were also increasing the frequency of eating and the quantity of what they ate. Consumers were happy, because now they could sit down in a restaurant and eat for hours for just one price. Entire families would converge on these restaurants almost as if it were a holiday and gorge on mounds of food until they literally couldn't shove any more in. In their minds, they were coming out ahead, because they ate three servings or more yet they only paid for one. Everyone seemed to win with these expanded portions and "can't beat" prices.

It's not surprising that as the number of eating establishments increased by 75 percent between 1977 and 1991,[2] there was at the same time a dramatic rise in the percentage of the population who were overweight or obese. Even more eateries have come into existence since 1991 and the average weight of both adults and children simply continue to rise to the point that we're at epidemic proportions. One well-reported study showed that the frequency of eating out, especially at fast-food restaurants, is associated with a higher body mass index (BMI).[3]

Restaurants are notoriously tricky for those who are trying to watch their calories and focus on healthy eating. The menu might give you the name of a dish and what's in it, but it's what the menu doesn't share with you that causes the problems. You often don't know how many ounces are in that steak, how much butter was used in that cream sauce, or how much mayonnaise was heaped on that sandwich. It's this lack of knowledge and loss of control that has made it difficult to maintain healthy eating standards away from home. In fact, over the last several decades, data has shown that we spend less time in our own kitchens and at our own dining room tables, and more time eating out where portion sizes and calorie counts are bound to be much too large. According to the U.S. Bureau of Labor Statistics, Consumer Expenditure Survey, the more money people make, the more they spend on food away from home.[4] Thankfully, several local and federal laws that require publishing nutritional information on menus or posters have been passed or are in the process of being passed. Consumers who are seeing calorie counts of their favorite foods are experiencing calorie sticker shock.

Let's take a quick walk down memory lane and look at how the portions we consume have spiraled out of control. These comparisons have been made available by the National Heart, Lung, and Blood Institute Obesity Education Initiative.

Calorie Counts

	20 Years Ago	Today	Difference
Bagel	140	350	210
Cheeseburger	333	590	257
Spaghetti and meatballs	500	1,025	525
French fries	210	610	400
Soda	85	250	165
Turkey sandwich	320	820	500

The portions have changed dramatically across almost every category of food and of course the caloric intake has also increased accordingly. See the chart below.

Calorie Counts		
20 Years Ago	**Today**	**Increase**
8 oz coffee with whole milk and sugar	16 oz mocha coffee (steamed whole milk, mocha syrup)	
45 calories	350 calories	305 calories
Muffin (1.5 oz)	Muffin (4 oz)	
210 calories	500 calories	290 calories
Pepperoni pizza (2 lg slices)	Pepperoni pizza (2 lg slices)	
500 calories	850 calories	350 calories
Chicken Caesar salad (1.5 cups)	Chicken Caesar Salad (3.5 cups)	
390 calories	790 calories	400 calories
Slice of cheesecake (3 oz)	Slice of cheesecake (7 oz)	
260 calories	640 calories	380 calories

We are so accustomed to sitting down to portions that are double and sometimes triple what we really should be eating that we don't even recognize the excess. Actually, ballooning portion sizes have the opposite effect. When restaurants or friends serve us an appropriately sized portion, we think they're skimping or being cheap. And it's not just restaurants that are serving us too much. Many of the snack foods and soft drinks you find in vending machines and grocery stores keep growing in size, with multiple servings packed into one package or bottle. What would help all of us—providers and consumers alike—is to get back to basics and have a true understanding of what a serving is and what a portion is. The two are very different and being able to discern one from the other can go a long way in helping us reduce our waistlines and improve our health.

Serving Size vs. Portion Size

My grandfather has a saying, "Understanding is one of the greatest things in the world." I think about his words when I think about how much all of us would benefit from a simple understanding of the quantity of food we actually consume versus what we should be consuming.

We've established how portions have grown out of control in the last couple of decades. But definitions are in order to better illustrate the common mistake we all make when we sit down to eat. A portion size is the amount of a single food item served on a single eating occasion. For example, if you sit down to dinner and order mashed potatoes, the amount of potatoes you are served is considered a portion size. This amount, of course, can vary drastically depending on where you're eating. One restaurant might serve you half a cup of mashed potatoes while another might serve a full cup. Both of them are considered to be a portion, since that's what was served, but you would compare them by simply saying that one portion size is bigger than another.

Many, unfortunately, confuse portion size with serving size. A serving size is a standardized unit of measuring foods—for example, an ounce or a cup. It doesn't change from restaurant to restaurant or home to home. A serving size for a particular food is always the same. Let's take a box of Entenmann's Original Recipe Chocolate Chip cookies (my brother's favorite) to make the point. The nutrition facts on the back of the box state that the serving size is 3 cookies. However, the package contains 11 servings. So when my brother sits down in front of his computer and chomps down half the box of cookies, the portion size he just consumed would've been about 16 cookies. However, the number of servings he just consumed would've been a little more than 5. Serving sizes were originally created to give us a guideline for how much of a particular food we were supposed to be eating at one sitting. But as you can see with my brother's chocolate chip cookie example, and I'm sure in your own life, you rarely consume *just* one serving of something. And to make matters even worse, manufacturers rarely include only one serving in a package or bottle or can. What you pick off the shelf or out of the cooler typically has 1.5, 2, 3, or even more servings. The problem is that most of us don't even think about looking at the labeling to see exactly how much we're consuming. We typically eat and drink all of the food or beverage item in one container as if it were meant to be consumed at one sitting.

Eating so much at one meal might not be a bad thing if we made the decision to eat fewer calories at subsequent meals. Let's say you have a really big lunch for some special occasion. One way to balance out your calorie intake would be to eat a small dinner that night. Unfortunately, this self-regulation proves difficult for many to do. In fact, some studies have found that people who ate larger portion sizes did not notice how big the portions were and went on to eat a normal amount of food at the following meal.[5] This excess calorie consumption is a perfect setup for weight gain.

Cheat Sheet for How Much to Eat

In a perfect world, every time we sat down to a meal we'd be provided with the ingredients in what we were about to eat as well as the appropriate serving sizes. This would make our life a lot easier when trying to figure out what to eat and how much of it to eat. Well, we don't live in a perfect world—far from it. So the best we can do is have a visual representation of what a serving looks like and apply that to the food we're served. Here's your cheat sheet when you need to make a fast decision.

Grains	Physical Equivalent
1 cup of cereal flakes	Baseball
1 plain pancake	Compact disc
1 slice of bread	Video cassette tape case
1/2 cup of cooked rice	Lightbulb
1/2 cup of cooked pasta	Lightbulb

Fruits & Vegetables	Physical Equivalent
1 baked potato	Computer mouse
1 cup of salad greens	Baseball
1/2 cup of grapes	About 16 small-medium grapes
1 medium fruit	Baseball
1 cup of cooked vegetables	Baseball
1 cup of strawberries	About 12 berries
1 cup carrots	12 baby carrots

Fats & Oils	Physical Equivalent
1 tablespoon oil	Poker chip
1 tablespoon mayonnaise	Poker chip
1 tablespoon salad dressing	Poker chip
1 tablespoon butter or spread	Poker chip

Meats, Fish & Nuts	Physical Equivalent
3 ounces grilled or baked fish	1 checkbook
3 ounces lean meat or poultry	Deck of cards
2 tablespoons peanut butter	Golf ball
2 tablespoons hummus	Golf ball
$1/4$ cup of pistachios	24 pistachios
$1/4$ cup of almonds	12 almonds

Dairy & Cheese	Physical Equivalent
$1/2$ cup of ice cream	Lightbulb
1 cup of yogurt	Baseball
$1^{1}/_{2}$ ounces cheese	3 stacked dice
$1/2$ cup frozen yogurt	Lightbulb

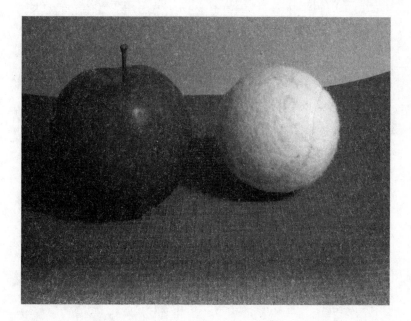

Fruits

One small apple is about the same size as a tennis ball and equals one fruit serving, or about 60 calories.

Other fruit servings:

Fruit	1 Serving (60 Calories)
Apple, sweetened	$1/3$ cup
Banana	1 small
Cherries	15 whole
Strawberries, whole	$1^1/_2$ cups
100 percent fruit juice, unsweetened	$1/2$ cup

Source: MayoClinic.com

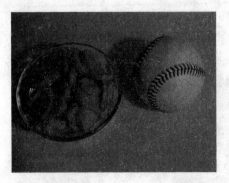

Cooked Carrots

Half a cup of cooked carrots is about the same as half a baseball and equals one vegetable serving—approximately 25 calories.

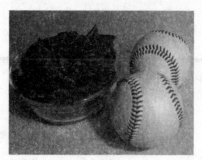

Raw Spinach

Two cups of raw leafy spinach are about the same as two baseballs and equals one vegetable serving—approximately 25 calories.

Other vegetable servings:

Vegetable	1 Serving (25 Calories)
Asparagus, cooked	6 spears ($1/2$ cup)
Cauliflower	1 cup florets (about 8)
Green beans, canned or frozen	$2/3$ cup
Tomato sauce, canned	$1/3$ cup
Zucchini, cooked or fresh	$3/4$ cup

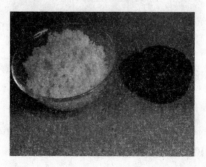

Carbohydrates: Brown Rice

One third of a cup of cooked brown rice is about the same size as a hockey puck and equals one carbohydrate serving—approximately 70 calories.

Other carbohydrate servings:

Carbohydrate	1 Serving (70 Calories)
Bagel, whole-grain	½ bagel (3" diameter)
Bun or roll, whole-grain	1 small
Cereal, cold, flake-type	¾ cup
Crackers, whole wheat	8
Muffin, any flavor	1 small

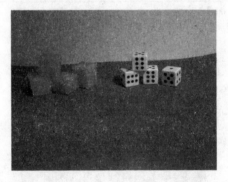

Dairy/Cheese

One and a half to 2 ounces of low-fat hard cheddar cheese is about the same size as three to four dice and equals one protein/dairy serving—approximately 110 calories.

Other dairy/cheese servings:

Protein/dairy	1 Serving (110 Calories)
Cheese, ricotta, part-skim	1/3 cup
Cheese, American	1.5 slices
Milk, skim or 1%	1 cup
Soy milk, low-fat	1 cup
Yogurt, plain, unsweetened	2/3 cup
Source: Mayoclinic.com	

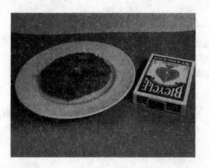

Protein/Dairy: Hamburger and More

A 3-ounce patty of cooked lean chop meat is about the same size as a deck of cards and equals one protein/dairy serving, or about 130 calories.

Fast Food on 500 Calories or Less

It's a fact of life that most people are going to routinely consume some amount of fast food. For some it might be once a week, for others, unfortunately, it might be once a day. Whatever the frequency, being smart about what foods you consume at a fast-food restaurant can make what is typically an unhealthy situation at least somewhat healthier.

Most fast-food restaurants have woken up to the cause and now offer a variety of foods in a variety of sizes that fall across the spectrum from really unhealthy to healthy. The problem is that too many people who consume fast food choose items that fall in the somewhat healthy to *really* unhealthy portion of the spectrum.

To make your task easier, here's a few of the most popular fast-food outlets and some examples of what you can get for 500 calories or less.

McDonald's

Menu Item	Number of Calories
Chicken McNuggets (4 pc), Apple Dippers with Low-Fat Caramel Dip, and 1% Low-Fat Milk Jug (8 fl oz)	390
McChicken Sandwich	360
Quarter Pounder	410
Filet-O-Fish	380
Premium Grilled Chicken Classic Sandwich	420
Ranch Snack Wrap	270
Honey Mustard Snack Wrap (grilled) and small French fries	490

Menu Item	Number of Calories
Premium Southwest Salad with Grilled Chicken with Newman's Own Low-Fat Family Recipe Italian Dressing	380
Egg McMuffin	300
Fruit 'n Yogurt Parfait	160

Burger King

Menu Item	Number of Calories
Double Cheeseburger	460
TENDERGRILL Chicken Sandwich	490
Ham Omelet Sandwich	290
KRAFT Macaroni and Cheese Kids Meal	160
TENDERGRILL Garden Salad (with Chicken)	460
Side Garden Salad with Ranch Dressing	330
Side Garden Salad with Light Italian Dressing	260
Medium Salted French Fries	440
VEGGIE Burger	420
Fresh Apple Fries	70

Wendy's

Menu Item	Number of Calories
Double Jr. Cheeseburger Deluxe	390
Small Fries	330
Value Fries	210
Grilled Chicken Go Wrap	250
Homestyle Chicken Fillet	470
Premium Fish Filet	500
5-piece Spicy Chicken Nuggets	230
Caesar, Side Salad (with Ranch dressing packet and croutons)	350
Mandarin Oranges	80
Small Vanilla Frosty	310

Arby's

Menu Item	Number of Calories
Roast Chicken Club Sandwich	460
Crispy Chicken Tenders (3 pieces)	360
Medium Roast Beef Sandwich	450
Ham & Swiss Melt Sandwich	300
Ham, Egg & Cheese Croissant	270
Bacon, Egg & Cheese Biscuit	450
Junior Roast Beef Sandwich with Apple Sauce and 1% Low-Fat White Milk	450

Menu Item	Number of Calories
Chopped Farmhouse Chicken Salad (grilled)	260
Chopped Italian Salad	390
Small Curly Fries	410

Subway

Menu Item	Number of Calories
6" Oven Roasted Chicken Sandwich	320
6" Sweet Onion Chicken Teriyaki Sandwich	380
Footlong Veggie Delite Sandwich	460
6" BLT Sandwich	360
6" Barbecue Chicken Sandwich	310
Oven Roasted Chicken (strips) Salad	130
Turkey Breast & Ham Salad	120
Egg White & Cheese Muffin	140
6" Black Forest Ham, Egg, & Cheese Omelet Sandwich	450
Hash Browns (4 pieces)	150

EAT Plan

◆ Divide your daily food intake into 4 small meals and 2 or 3 snacks. This will help you control your portions. Try to keep each meal around 500 calories or less if you're trying to lose weight and 600 calories or less if you're trying to maintain weight.

◆ Eat a fist. Try to make your food portion sizes no bigger than your fist. If you have a large fist, then use three quarters of your fist as a visual guide. Each meal except for breakfast should contain two fists of vegetables. Always try to get in one serving of fruit with breakfast. Freshly squeezed juice or fruit smoothies counts as fruit.

◆ Eat from a salad plate instead of the normally large dinner plates. Make sure half of your plate is covered with low-calorie vegetables.

You Are What You Drink 8

- ✦ The Miracle of Water
- ✦ Floating Calories
- ✦ Drinking Fat
- ✦ The Buzz of Energy Drinks
- ✦ Your Personal Drink Chart

America has a drinking problem and doesn't know it. On a daily basis we guzzle beverages in excessive amounts. But while many of them taste great, they are full of empty calories that carry no nutritional value. Most people can identify the dangers of fried foods and fat-laden snacks, but when it comes to understanding the liquids we drink and their potential health implications, many are either in denial or truly drowning in a river of ignorance. What we drink is just as important as what we eat. Choosing the right drinks not only means you can quench your thirst, but it also means that you can potentially decrease your risk for disease, increase your success at losing weight, and improve the quality of your life. Choosing the wrong drinks and indulging them in excess can be a recipe for disaster. What most people don't understand is that while the old adage "you are what you eat" remains as relevant as ever, it's every bit as much true that "you are what you drink."

Water

In the beginning all we had was water. No coffee, soda, juices, or energy drinks, just pure water. It was and still is enough to replenish the fluids we lose on a daily basis and keep us hydrated. For thousands of years, water was all we relied on to keep our body's fluid balance at proper levels. Our bodies are estimated to be about 60 to 70 percent water. It's everywhere—in our blood, muscles, lungs, and brain. Without water, we wouldn't be able to live. It's necessary for some of the body's most critical functions, including transporting oxygen to cells, removing wastes, regulating body temperature, helping nutrients reach needy organs, and protecting our joints and organs.

Water is abundant in our environment: the U.S. Geological Survey estimates that about 70 percent of the earth is covered with water— that a total of approximately 332 million cubic miles. However, 97 percent of this water is not drinkable because it's saltwater, leaving only 3 percent of the world's water as freshwater and suitable for drinking. This still amounts to enough water to nourish our bodies and support our existence.

We constantly lose water—every second of the day—through sweating, breathing, and voiding. So how much water should we be taking in each day to replenish what we lose? Conventional wisdom has said eight cups (64 ounces) a day, but the truth is that no one really knows where that number comes from. When the idea of eight cups started making its rounds many years ago, there was no real scientific evidence to support it. But the truth is that it's next to impossible to predict how much water any given person needs each day. Our needs are as varied as the color of our eyes and the texture of our hair.

Spice Up Your Water

Squeeze in big chunks of juicy fruit then dunk them in

Citrus Splash: add slices of lemon, lime, orange, or grapefruit;
  sometimes try more than one

Thinly slice a cucumber and add it to your water

Add a few dashes of mint

Refrigerate seltzer water and add raspberries or sliced strawberries

Tap Water vs. Bottled Water

The debate about tap water versus bottled water has been going on for a painfully long time. Unfortunately, greed, politics, and other agendas have gotten in the way of an unbiased declaration of the truth. Thousands of medical papers have been written, analyses proffered, and expertise proclaimed, all in the interest of deciding what the best source is for our water.

After reading numerous reports and studying very dull, but at times informative analyses, it appears to me that the benefits of bottled water are overblown and can mostly be chalked up to extremely clever marketing. Bottled water is a multibillion-dollar industry, largely driven by marketing that plays on the fears of consumers. If you were to believe the claims of bottled water manufacturers, you would think that tap water was full of impurities that could adversely affect your health. The truth, however, is very different. Numerous unbiased studies have shown that most of the tap water in this country is clean and completely suitable for drinking without any threat to our health. Ironically, some studies have shown that some bottled water actually contains contaminants and higher-than-desired levels of arsenic.

Strictly from a health and economic perspective, drinking tap water is completely fine. Slick marketing and pretty commercials try to make you think that water collected from pristine glaciers has a superior quality, but the truth is that billions of dollars could be saved if consumers would realize that this dramatically more expensive water had no real benefits, except for maybe its convenience.

Tips for Adding Water to Your Diet

◆ Get into the habit: Just like you start and end your day by brushing your teeth, bookend your day with a glass of water.

◆ Drink one cup of water at each meal. If you eat 3 meals a day and you bookend your day with water as suggested above, then you've easily consumed 5 cups of water without even trying.

◆ Fresh lemonade is another way to get in your daily water requirement. Just squeeze some lemons and combine with water and make sure you minimize the added sugar.

◆ Pack your water and take it with you. Get a quart or half-gallon container and add a couple of slices of lemon or cucumber. Refrigerate the water and when heading to work or out for the day, carry your container with you so that you can sip all day.

Hidden Calories

When it comes to packing on those unwanted pounds, excess calories in liquids produce the same result as excess calories in food: weight gain. Unfortunately, too many people think either that liquids don't contain calories or that the calories contained in liquids are less fattening. Both are miles from the truth and, combined with how easy it is to down big quantities while barely noticing, have led people to thoughtlessly drink beverages full of hidden calories.

Below is a listing of some very popular drinks and the surprising amount of calories they contain.

Beverage (8 Ounces or 1 Cup)	Calories
Soda (nondiet)	110
Whole milk	150
2% low-fat milk	120
1% low-fat milk	100
Fat-free milk	90
Soy milk	100
Orange juice	110
Apple juice (from concentrate)	110
Cranberry juice cocktail	140
Coffee, black, plain brewed	2
Coffee with cream (2 tablespoons half-and-half)	20
Coffee with heavy whipping cream (2 tablespoon)	52
Coffee, caffè mocha with 2% milk	130

continued

Beverage (8 Ounces or 1 Cup)	Calories
Coffee, Peppermint White	240
Canada Dry Mandarin Orange Seltzer water (8 oz)	0
Schweppes Tonic Water (8 oz)	90
Lipton Iced Tea with Lemon (20 oz)	200
Vitamin Water (formula 50)	50
Nantucket Nectars (Grapeade)	130
Bud Light (12 ounces)	110
Red Bull (12 ounces)	160
Gatorade Thirst Quencher (32 ounces)	200

One of the dangerous qualities of liquid calories is that they behave differently from solid food calories in one important way. When you eat a solid meal, your stomach starts to physically fill up with the food and your stomach stretches. This stretching sends a message to the brain that you've eaten enough and you get a feeling of "satiety," or fullness. You no longer have the urge to consume more food. Also, the intestines release nerve regulators and hormones that help you feel full. Liquids don't operate the same way. There has been strong scientific evidence that our bodies don't detect the calories in liquids the same way they do with solid foods. Liquids can quench our thirst and tell our bodies that we no longer desire something to drink, but when it comes to satisfying our hunger, liquid calories do a very poor job. Because liquids travel more quickly than food through the intestinal tract, they decrease the speed with which nutrients are absorbed and this can affect the "feel-full" hormones and nerve signals.

The danger in all of this comes with the extra calories the beverages bring. You can sit down and drink several hundred calories in liquids, and still eat the same amount of solid food that you would've eaten had you not drunk the beverages. So you are not only consuming calories in the solid food, but now you're adding extra calories with the beverages. Most people don't think about these calories when they're monitoring their calorie counts, and over time this could lead to unexpected weight gain. Take the simple example of someone who drinks a couple of 12-ounce sodas each day. On average these sodas contain 150 calories. Drinking two or three of them each day can be enough calories added to your diet to gain a pound in just one week. And for many, 16-ounce sodas have become the norm. If this consumption rate continues, and our lack of physical activity continues to decrease, it won't be a pretty picture.

Just because there are hidden calories in a variety of beverages, it doesn't mean you can't occasionally imbibe some of the less healthy, more calorie-rich products. What it means is that you should be aware of these calories and drink these beverages in moderation. Is a soda every once in a while going to have a negative impact on your health? Absolutely not. But if you are guzzling three sodas a day and practicing other unhealthy behaviors, then that's a completely different story.

Coffee and Tea

Water is, thankfully, the most consumed beverage in the United States and around the world. Right behind water consumption comes tea and coffee. In 2009 alone, Americans consumed well over 60 billion servings of tea, 82 percent of it black tea and 17 percent of it green tea. On any given day, about one half of the American population drinks tea.[1] Coffee is not as popular as tea but we still drink a lot, with the average consumption among coffee drinkers being approximately three cups per day.[2]

When tea is consumed plain without sweetener, milk, or other things mixed in, it is virtually calorie free. Tea is nearly 5,000 years old. It first became popular throughout Europe and the American colonies in the 1600s. It has been very popular in Europe ever since, and over the last couple of decades, its popularity has continued to increase here in the United States. A lot of the recent interest in tea has been because of the health benefits that many manufacturers and health advocates have suggested are contained in the brewed leaves.

Tea has a purity that few other beverages have. It doesn't contain fat, sodium, sugar, or carbonation. It does, however, contain flavonoids, which are natural, biologically active substances that have antioxidant properties. Antioxidants are important to our health as they can fight against the free radicals in our bodies that, over time, can cause damage and lead to chronic disease. While everything is not yet known about tea's health-promoting properties, there has been an onslaught of recent studies that suggest its impact. For example, one Harvard study found that people who drank a cup or more of black tea each day reduced their risk of heart attack by 44 percent.[3] In a study conducted by the U.S. Department of Agriculture, participants who drank five cups of black tea per day along with a diet moderately low in fat and cholesterol reduced their LDL cholesterol (the bad type) by about 6 to 10 percent after three weeks.[4]

The debate surrounding coffee's impact on health has been much more controversial. When consumed plain it, too, doesn't have any calories. But there has been a long-running debate about caffeine. Following the reports and studies regarding coffee's long-term health effects can be confusing and frustrating; there is no consensus about what is safe and what can cause adverse effects. For every study that's published concluding drinking too much caffeinated coffee can be harmful, there's one that suggests the benefits of the flavonoids it contains outweigh the potential harm caused by caffeine.

One thing that experts do, however, agree upon is how drinking some coffee concoctions can contribute significantly to weight gain. For example, a Starbucks 12-ounce Peppermint White Chocolate Mocha with 2% milk and whipped cream contains 420 calories. This is more calories than many people consume in an entire breakfast. But beyond the excessive amount of calories, there's more bad news. This single drink contains 15 grams of fat and 61 grams of carbohydrates—*61 grams!* That's the equivalent of 14.5 teaspoons of sugar!

So how many cups of coffee should one consume per day? There is no perfect answer. Coffee is not a "required" drink, nor is it considered to be a drink that has a tremendous positive impact on your health. Drinking too much coffee can cause a person to become jittery and in some instances even increase the heart rate. Caffeine's stimulation of the central nervous system can be uncomfortable. Some experts suggest drinking three or four cups of coffee per day is fine, but this number may not apply to everyone, especially those who might have heart conditions or central nervous system problems. Just the same, a chronic coffee drinker can also run into problems when trying to cut back, in some cases experiencing symptoms of caffeine withdrawal such as headaches, irritability, restlessness, muscle stiffness, and poor concentration. It's not the coffee bean that's the issue, it's all the trendy things added to the coffee that are problems.

Juice

Be smart when it comes to juice. If chosen and prepared correctly, juice can be an extremely healthy component in your diet. It can contain a bonanza of vitamins and other nutrients that have a positive impact on your overall well-being. Juice is most healthful in its most natural state. Freshly squeezed juice, while typically more expensive than other "processed" juice, is the best way to drink up those amazing nutrients as well as to answer any craving for sweets. You might not get exactly the same benefits you get from eating fruit, but if that's not possible, then freshly squeezed juice is the next best thing. One of the most important aspects of fresh juice is that no sugars are added; the natural collection of sugars already found in the fruit give you the sweet kick you desire.

Problems arise, however, when you start drinking juices that are not "all natural," but instead are loaded with added sugars, artificial preservatives, and other additives. Look carefully at the label to reveal these less desirable drinks. Red flags should go up when you see phrases such as: "from concentrate," "juice drink," "juice blend," "juice cocktail." Concentrated juice means that fresh orange juice has undergone a vaporization process where the water is extracted from the juice; what remains is frozen. When you want to drink the juice, you thaw the concentrate, add water, and drink. Sometimes concentrated juices have sugars added to them in the process and sometimes they don't. You will have to read the ingredient label to see.

Terms such as "juice drink," "juice blend," and "juice cocktail" are a clear indication that this is *not* a 100 percent juice beverage. There is *some* fruit juice in these products, but there could be as little as 10 percent and the rest of the beverage is made up of sugar, flavoring, and other additives. If possible, reduce your consumption of these "quasi-juice" forms. Not only are you missing out on the true benefits of juice, but many of these products contain a tremendous number of calories, as much as 260 calories in one serving. Unfortunately, when most people see the word "juice" they jump to the conclusion that the drink in question is healthy and full of important nutrients. Not so fast. The overall quality truly depends on the percentage of fruit juice the beverage contains and whether or not sugars have been added in processing. The terms "freshly squeezed" or "made from freshly squeezed" are the phrases that you should be looking for when selecting your juice.

Alcohol

Throughout the thousands of years that humans have consumed spirits there's been a lively debate about alcohol's benefits and detriments. It seems every year brings a new study trying to resolve how much, if any, alcohol we should consume. We do know that alcohol has two faces, and which one you see depends on the dose. The source of alcohol's potency can be found in a rather simple molecule called ethanol that can impact the body in many different ways. It can have a direct influence on several organs and systems, including the brain, heart, liver, stomach, gallbladder, cholesterol and triglyceride levels, levels of insulin, inflammation, and blood clotting.

Research has made it very clear that drinking alcohol is like climbing a slippery slope. If you imbibe the right kind of alcohol in modest portions, then you might reap some health benefits. If you overindulge, however, you are at risk for severe complications. By no means do experts advocate that people drink alcohol for its potential benefits. If you are not a drinker, the healthier choice is to stay that way. However, if you do find yourself wanting to enjoy a spirit now and again, the key is to do so in moderation. Studies vary in their conclusions about how helpful moderate drinking can be to your health, and there can even be differences in health benefits between two people who drink the same type and amount of alcohol. Red wine has long been touted for its heart-healthy positive impact, but doctors aren't completely sure about the specific ingredient(s) that might deliver the benefit. Many have touted the benefits of antioxidants such as flavonoids and resveratrol. Some believe that these antioxidants work by increasing the level of "good cholesterol" (HDL) and protecting against artery damage.

Some studies have shown that moderate alcohol consumption can:

- Lower your risk for gallstones
- Reduce your risk for strokes
- Reduce your risk for heart disease
- Reduce your risk from dying of a heart attack
- Lower your risk for type 2 diabetes

So what is moderate consumption? There are several definitions depending on the source, but typically scientists define it as one drink per day for women and one to two drinks per day for men. This is how the Mayo Clinic's Web site defines moderate drinking:

Healthy men 66 and older: a maximum of 3 drinks per occasion or 7 drinks per week
Healthy men 65 and younger: a maximum of 4 drinks per occasion or 14 drinks per week
Healthy women: a maximum of 3 drinks per occasion or 7 drinks per week

Examples of "one drink" include:

Beer: 12 ounces (355 milliliters)
Wine: 5 ounces (148 milliliters)
80-proof distilled spirits 1.5 ounces (44 milliliters)

One big misperception is that if you don't drink all week, you can save up and splurge on the weekends. *Wrong!* Not only will you find yourself quite inebriated, but there are absolutely no health benefits when you overindulge; in fact, just the opposite effect will be achieved.

The dangers of high-volume, long-term alcohol consumption certainly outweigh its potential but not guaranteed benefits. It's because of this vast array of complications that experts recommend either abstention from alcohol or drinking in moderation. While most people know that alcohol can damage the liver and increase your risk for heart disease, there's a long list of other potential complications that might raise your eyebrows.

Dangers of Excessive Alcohol Consumption

High blood pressure

Stroke

Heart disease

Cirrhosis (scarring) of the liver

Certain cancers (breast, mouth, throat, esophagus, liver, colon, and rectal)

Pancreatitis

Miscarriage

Health damage to unborn child

Suicide

Addiction

Accidental serious injury or death

Sudden death in those who already have cardiovascular disease

The bottom line is that alcohol should be consumed in moderation. Drinking socially and occasionally tends not to present problems. You have to know your own body and reaction to alcohol. If you are already at risk for illness, it's likely that alcohol will only complicate and increase your risk. If you find yourself unable to stop at a few drinks and needing to drink yourself into reckless intoxication, then you need to consider whether the potential dangers are really worth it. Alcohol has been around for thousands of years. It can be enjoyed like other beverages in the proper balance.

Energy Drinks

In this fast-paced world in which we now live, with technology such as BlackBerries and Facebook keeping us connected around the clock, there's an even greater desire to increase our energy levels and alertness. In the past, this boost of energy was achieved through caffeinated drinks or soda as well as stimulants in the form of pills, many of which are considered illegal. Then in the mid-1980s an Austrian entrepreneur by the name of Dietrich Mateschitz and a Thai national named Chaleo Yoovidhya adapted the Thai energy drink Krating Daeng into Red Bull and sold it in Asia and Europe with great success. In 1997, it was introduced to the United States and since its launch it has become the bestselling energy drink in the world.

Red Bull literally created an industry, one that is now valued at billions of dollars and will likely continue to grow as new energy drinks hit the market every year with promises to reinvigorate users and increase alertness. Their aggressive marketing has made all kinds of claims, including increasing concentration and reaction speed, improving mood, stimulating metabolism, and improving performance.

Most energy drinks are carbonated and contain significant amounts of caffeine and sugar. Other prominent ingredients include amino acids such as taurine, herbal stimulants such as guarana, and B vitamins. Some of these drinks contain as much as 80 milligrams of caffeine per can, almost the same amount found in a cup of brewed coffee and twice the amount of that found in a cup of tea.

Energy drinks have become particularly popular in bars and nightclubs, where consumers mix the energy drink with alcohol hoping that the stimulating effect of the caffeine in the energy drink will counteract the depressant effect of the alcohol, thus keeping them wider awake and more alert as they move into drunkenness. The most popular combination has been Red Bull and vodka. The Red Bull deceives drinkers into thinking they are not impaired, and this leads them to drink more and reach extremely high blood alcohol levels. As you can imagine, with names like Monster Energy, Full Throttle Energy, and Rockstar Energy, these drinks are heavily marketed to a younger, partying clientele.

Experts are not convinced that these manufacturers' claims are true, but there are even bigger questions surrounding the negative health consequences of constant use of these drinks. One of the most prevalent concerns is the number of calories in these drinks. Energy drinks purport to give their boost via the typically large amounts of caffeine they contain, but they also are loaded with sugar, which drives up the calorie counts. Take a look at some popular energy drinks and the amount of calories packed inside each can.

Beverage (per 12 Ounces)	Number of Calories
Red Bull	160
Monster (original)	150
Rockstar (original)	210
Full Throttle (citrus)	165
Sobe Adrenaline Rush (Taurine)	195
Sobe No Fear (Super Energy)	195
Amp	165
Rib It	195

Health experts are most concerned because there have been relatively few scientific studies that have looked at the health effects of these drinks and the potential dangers posed by mixing them with other substances. Caffeine is a known stimulant, but so are some of the other ingredients often used in energy drinks, such as taurine and guarana.

What effect does combining these ingredients have on the nervous system? Some experts believe that consumers are at risk for such symptoms as heart palpitations, irritability, sleeping difficulty, anxiety, indigestion, and blood pressure changes. If you're looking for an immediate boost of energy, think twice before you reach for that can of liquid caffeinated candy. There are safer and more proven ways to kick up your energy, whether it's sports drinks, green or black tea, fruit juices, water, or even low-fat milk.

Soda

America leads the international pack when it comes to soda consumption. According to the Global Marketing Information Database, Americans consume more than 57 gallons of soft drinks in a single year. This puts us way ahead of second-place Ireland (33 gallons) and third-place Canada and Norway (32 gallons). Excessive consumption has been widely implicated in the country's dramatic rise in obesity over the last decade, especially in children. Many studies have looked at the rise in sugary drink consumption and correlated it to the country's expanding waistlines.

While the negative consequences of soda consumption can be fairly debated, there's very little argument anyone can make about soda actually being beneficial to your health except that diet soda is better than regular soda when attempting to lose weight. Most 12-ounce cans of soda contain 150 to 160 calories. The good news is that U.S. consumption of soda has decreased over the last eleven years, with new figures putting consumption at 22 percent less than our peak consumption back in 1998. Experts believe several factors have played a role in this reduction including health campaigns, the acknowledged link with obesity, low-carb diets, the ban on soft drinks in some schools, and the rising popularity of bottled water.

While it's easy to point a finger at sodas and blame them for the continuing rise in obesity, the truth is that consumers are at the very least equally to blame. Consuming a couple of cans of soda each week should not have any substantive impact on our waistlines or health, but the problem is one of portion control. Moderation is the key when it comes to consuming soft drinks just as it is when eating foods that are higher in calories and lower in nutritional value. If you're trying to lose weight, cutting back on sodas can be of some benefit, as can drinking diet sodas that don't have any calories. But ultimately it's about balance and not overindulging. Drinking soda in moderation is not harmful when you practice healthy behaviors such as exercise.

Diet Soda

Diet sodas can be quite beneficial to those trying to lose weight for one reason: they contain no calories and thus do not add to your daily caloric consumption. The caveat, however, is that people who drink diet soda are sometimes mistaken in their belief that saving calories with their diet drink means that they can increase calories elsewhere. The diet drinker's logic is simple: *If I were to drink three cans of regular soda over the course of the day, that would mean I'd be consuming almost 500 calories. But since I'm drinking diet soda instead, that means I'm saving 500 calories. Now I can consume those calories elsewhere, such as in snacks or eating bigger portions during my meals.*

Yes, you would be saving 500 calories by drinking the diet soda; the problem is the second half of the argument. Switching the calorie savings to greater food consumption is a critical mistake. Most people don't know how to count calories, and when making the switch, end up eating not just the 500 calories they saved, but actually eating more. So you go from saving the calories by drinking the diet soda to actually eating more calories than you would have had you simply had the regular soda. Don't use calorie transfers to compensate for your diet soda savings.

Another caution regarding diet soda is that it actually increases your appetite for calories. This sounds strange on the face of it, especially since diet soda is supposed to eliminate calories from your diet. Well, it does in the strict sense that it doesn't contain calories; however, several studies have suggested that zero-calorie artificial sweeteners can cause the body to crave more calories, often in the form of carbohydrates and sugar.[5] If your body strongly says "I want more calories," your inclination may be to find those calories in a Danish, cookies, chips—whatever will give you a quick burst of calories. So while you're saving calories by drinking diet soda instead of regular soda, you can easily end up defeating your efforts by consuming extra calories in other foods. The bottom line is that if you're going to drink diet soda, don't increase your calorie intake in other parts of your diet.

Your Drink Chart

The famous food pyramid created by the USDA has been a guiding force in our daily nutritional habits and recommendations since it was created. Dividing up the major food categories has helped us create a balanced approach to eating, which ensures we are consuming the right amount of the various nutrients our bodies need. But what about beverages? A group of nutrition experts from across the U.S. formed the independent Beverage Guidance Panel, whose stated mission is to provide guidance on the relative health and nutritional benefits and risks of various beverage categories. The panel presented its advice in a six-level pitcher similar to the classic food pyramid. Just as in the food pyramid, the lower the level, the greater the percentage of that type of beverage should appear in your diet plan. Water is at the very bottom,

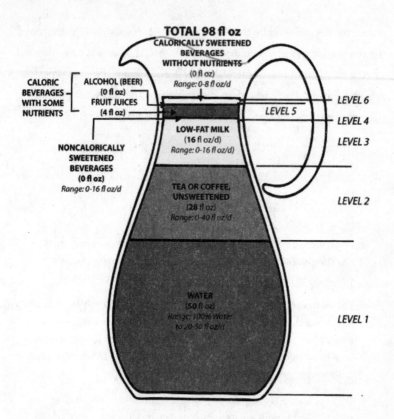

Suggested beverage consumption pattern for a person who requires 2,200 calories per day, providing 10 percent of calories from beverages. The values 50, 28, 16, and 4 fl oz are shown for illustrative purposes only; the total consumption should sum to 98 fl oz, as shown at the top of the figure. The range listed at each level refers to the Beverage Guidance Panel's suggested consumption range for each beverage. Caffeine is a limiting factor for coffee and tea consumption; consume up to 400 mg per day, or approximately 32 fl oz of coffee (can replace water). Noncalorically sweetened beverages can substitute for tea and coffee with the same limitations regarding caffeine, up to 16 fl oz per day (this is adapted from the Beverage Guidance Panel's original recommendation of up to 32 fl oz per day). (Adapted with permission from *Am. J. Clin. Nutr.* (2006; 83:529–42), © American Society for Nutrition.)

which means it should be the dominant liquid in your diet. At the top of the pitcher are those beverages, such as alcohol, that should be consumed in very small amounts. Remember, this is just a guide. No one is perfect, nor can anyone be expected to eat and drink perfectly, but following these guidelines as closely as possible can make a big difference.

EAT Plan

✦ Water should be 50 percent of your day's beverage consumption. You can certainly mix plain water with a couple of cups of flavored water if you like, but remember that flavored water contains calories.

✦ Cut whatever amount of soda you typically drink in half. Try to reduce your soda consumption to 12 ounces per day. Remember, the key is moderation. While soda isn't the healthiest of drinks, you can certainly still enjoy it, just make it the smallest portion of your nonalcoholic beverage intake.

✦ Try to consume 1 cup of freshly squeezed juice each day. It might be inconvenient to squeeze it yourself, but many stores and even smaller delis typically have freshly squeezed juice available. Yes, it's definitely more expensive than the reconstituted concentrated juices, but the extra cash is worth the nutritional purity you'll be drinking and the added sugars and preservatives that you'll be avoiding. Remember, spending a little extra now means saving a lot later when you avoid many of the illnesses that come with long-term consumption of unhealthy beverages.

Unearthing the "Organic" Truth

9

- ✦ The Real Meaning of Organic
- ✦ Be a Label Hound
- ✦ Beware of Organic Hype
- ✦ The Dirty Dozen

For a long time, whenever I saw the word "organic," three questions came immediately to mind: First, what in the heck does organic really mean? Second, are organic foods *really* healthier or is it just some great marketing ploy? Third, why are organic foods more expensive than those grown through conventional farming methods? I've come to learn that I'm far from being alone in asking these questions. Millions of others—and it's likely you're included in those millions—continue to ask the same questions. What's even more confusing is that when you search for these answers you have to be mindful of the source that provides them, because so many have a financial stake in this growing multibillion-dollar industry.

I'm not a farmer, conventional or organic, nor am I a food retailer. In other words, I don't have a horse in this race. I went on a mission to get the real answers not just for myself but for you as well. Here's what I found.

What Does Organic Mean?

Unlike some other terms in the food world, "organic" is not one that is supposed to be left open to interpretation. The term and when it should be used to describe food are clearly defined and surprisingly easy to understand. Here's the USDA definition:

ORGANIC MEAT, POULTRY, EGGS, AND DAIRY PRODUCTS COME FROM ANIMALS THAT ARE GIVEN NO ANTIBIOTICS OR GROWTH HORMONES. ORGANIC FOOD IS PRODUCED WITHOUT USING MOST CONVENTIONAL PESTICIDES; FERTILIZERS MADE WITH SYNTHETIC INGREDIENTS OR SEWAGE SLUDGE; BIOENGINEERING; OR IONIZING RADIATION. ORGANIC FOOD IS PRODUCED BY FARMERS WHO EMPHASIZE THE USE OF RE-NEWABLE RESOURCES AND THE CONSERVATION OF SOIL AND WATER TO ENHANCE ENVIRONMENTAL QUALITY FOR FUTURE GENERATIONS.

It takes quite a bit of work for manufacturers to be granted the right to use an organic label on food products. A government-approved certifier first has to inspect the farm where the food is grown to confirm that the farm is abiding by and meeting all of the rules necessary to meet USDA organic standards. Going even a step beyond the farmers, companies that handle or process organic food in preparation for supermarket shelves or restaurants must also be certified. Animals grown on organic farms eat organically grown feed, aren't confined 100 percent of the time (as they sometimes are on conventional farms), and aren't pumped with hormones or antibiotics. Many farms that might be using organic methods don't subscribe to the official certification, because it can be an onerous and expensive process.

Organic farming is quite different from conventional farming in both style and substance. The original purpose of organic farming was to encourage soil and water conservation and reduce pollution. In other words, it was an environmental preservation movement—a way of farming that still yielded the food we need to survive, but didn't ruin the land, air, or water in the process. Organic farmers don't use conventional methods to fertilize, control weeds, or prevent their livestock from becoming infected and developing disease (such as the mad cow disease, which is caused by prions, disease-causing proteins). A conventional farmer applies chemical fertilizers to promote plant growth whereas an organic farmer uses natural fertilizers such as manure or compost to feed the soil and plants. Conventional farmers spray insecticides to reduce pests and disease, while organic farmers use specially selected insects and birds, mating disruption or traps to reduce pests and disease. Conventional farmers use chemical herbicides to manage weeds, but organic farmers rotate crops, till the soil, hand weed, and mulch to better manage weeds.

In many ways, organic farming is a return to the old days of conventional farming, when chemicals and antibiotics weren't used on crops and animals. Farmers worked the land with their hands with great effort long before the invention of pesticides and chemical fertilizers that are now practically ubiquitous. But as the need for increased output grew and farms continued to battle bad weather, disease, and spoilage, farmers developed and adopted methods that would sustain and improve their crops and eventually increase or at least maintain their profits.

The use of pesticides, antibiotics, and chemicals in our food chain has recently been met with great resistance and controversy, and for good reason. Well-documented studies as well as common sense tell us that too many of these chemicals in our foods can have deleterious effects on our health and the environment. This push for safer and less destructive farming methods has led to a significant rise in organic farming across the world. According to the Economic Research Service of the USDA, "organic farming has been one of the fastest growing segments of U.S. agriculture for over a decade." When Congress passed the Organic Foods Production Act (OFPA) of 1990 there was less than a million acres of certified organic farmland. By 2002, certified organic farmland had doubled. In just the short three years between 2002 and 2005 there was another doubling. According to USDA data, the organic livestock business grew even faster. California remains the leading state in certified organic farmland, counting over 430,000 acres.

Know Your Labels

The Organic Foods Production Act required the USDA to develop national standards for organically produced agricultural products to assure consumers that products marketed as organic met consistent, uniform standards. A series of rules that govern marketing and production of organic products were established through the years with the final rule going into effect on October 21, 2002. As part of this final rule, the National Organic Program (NOP) defined requirements for labeling products as organic and as containing organic ingredients. In the case of organic food labeling, the words used actually make a big difference. Don't just look at the word "organic" and assume that product is made just like others that also have the word "organic" on their packages. It's important that you know the differences so that you can make the best choice and get the most for your money. Following are the established labeling standards and the USDA Organic seal that you should look for when shopping for certified products.

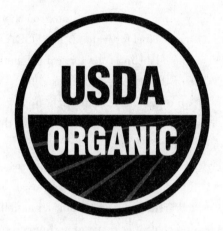

USDA Organic Seal

100 percent organic: These products must contain only organically produced ingredients. Manufacturers are allowed to display the USDA organic seal on these products.

Organic: These products must consist of at least 95 to 99 percent organically produced ingredients by weight. The remaining ingredients are not available organically but have been approved by NOP. Manufacturers are allowed to display the USDA organic seal on these products.

Made with organic ingredients: These are processed products that contain at least 70 percent organic ingredients. They are allowed to list up to three of the organic ingredients or food groups on the principal display panel. However, they don't meet the USDA threshold of 95 percent, so the organic seal *cannot* be used anywhere on the package.

Organic meat, poultry, eggs, and dairy products come from animals that are given no antibiotics or growth hormones.

Regardless of what you might see in the store, you should know that there is no official organic label for seafood. The USDA is still discussing how to create organic-labeling rules for seafood, but it's proving to be challenging. One of the biggest challenges is figuring out how to ensure that fish eat an organic diet. You might be able to accomplish this with farm-raised fish, but how do you guarantee this in wild fish that freely roam the waters?

You are likely to see other organic-sounding terms on food labels, but it's important that you don't get them confused. Remember, organic farming and food retailing have become a multibillion-dollar industry with increasing consumer demand and more producers trying to get their share of the profits. You will come across all kinds of marketing schemes intended to make you think you're buying something that you really aren't. Don't be tricked. Phrases such as "all-natural," "free-range," and "hormone-free" are commonly used by manufacturers to give you more information about the attributes of the products or the process they underwent while being grown or manufactured. But none of these terms means organic, nor are they a substitute for the word "organic." Unfortunately, too many consumers are confused by these healthy-sounding descriptive terms and erroneously think they are synonyms for organic. Certainly the manufacturers won't be too upset if you make that mistake. But now that you are informed, you won't!

It's Expensive to Be Organic

Given the claims and advantages that have been touted for organic foods, it's no wonder that so many people want to give organic a try. But when you stand in the produce section of your local supermarket and look at a display of blueberries that cost $4.99 per package and sitting right next to it looking exactly the same are regular blueberries just like your grandma used to buy at $2.50 a package, it makes you wonder why the organic price is higher. As a skeptical consumer, I had my doubts about the justification for charging higher prices, sometimes as much as 20 to 100 percent higher than conventionally grown products. Then I started digging around and most of it started to make sense.

It all supposedly starts with the farming. It's the old axiom: the more expensive a product is to produce, the higher the price a consumer must pay at retail. You'll get very little argument against the statement that organic farming tends to be more labor-intensive than conventional farming. Where conventional farmers can use herbicides to kill weeds, organic farmers can't. Their solution? Hand-picking the weeds, rotating the crops, and tilling the land. All three of these require manual labor, which means more costs in wages, which means a costlier crop once it's harvested. This is very different from producing designer handbags. Many of these so-called luxury handbags that sell for hundreds and thousands of dollars are manufactured in overseas warehouses where the labor is embarrassingly cheap and the work conditions are relatively inhumane. The mind-blowing markup that consumers pay by the time these handbags hit the shelves certainly can't be justified by the cost-of-labor argument. But in the case of organic products, the argument is quite relevant.

The next issue is one of scale. Organic farms tend to be much smaller than conventional farms. This causes a price increase in several ways. First, the smaller the farm, the smaller the crop you harvest, the higher your price to cover the fixed expenses of running the farm. A larger farm can have a larger crop harvest and charge a smaller amount for its products because the profit is made not by margins (how much charged per item versus what it actually cost to produce it), but volume (sell more at a lower cost and still make money because the volume of sales is so high). Also, it's important to look at the yield. No farm harvests and sells 100 percent of the crops it plants and grows or the animals it raises for slaughter. Whether it's disease, spoilage, weather, or that the crop/animal just doesn't make it, there is a certain amount of loss expected with each harvest. This loss is particularly high for organic farms, because they rely on natural and manual remedies and preventive methods rather than chemicals that are cheaper and often more effective on a larger scale. Where conventional farmers might expect a harvest loss of 10 percent, organic farmers can expect anywhere from 20 to 40 percent.

Organic certification guidelines also impose a certain amount of expense. Workers must be knowledgeable and skilled in specific methods so they can implement the necessary procedures, protocols, and changes to ensure the farm is in compliance with the required federal standards. Then you need a knowledgeable manager to make sure the workers are following the correct methods and everything is according to code. All of this requires manpower—and manpower equals money. While there are set guidelines for both conventional and organic farming, it's the organic farmers who have the highest bar to reach and stiffer requirements to meet.

Retail 101 teaches that "the slower the line moves, the more retailers will charge." Regardless of whether a product is organic or conventional, there's limited shelf space for food products. Retailers are in the business of making money, not making friends. If a line of products is selling more slowly than others, then they are left with the decision to either drop the line or charge more for it. Increasing the pricing means that even though they are moving fewer products, they can still make some kind of profit. It's all about the retail margin game. Many retailers say that while demand for organic food products has increased dramatically over the last several years, the vast majority of people still spend most of their money on conventional products. To make up for this difference in rate of sales, they sometimes increase the cost of organic foods even more to prevent losing money on the merchandise that doesn't sell.

Whether you agree or not, there are legitimate reasons why organic foods tend to be pricier than those that are conventionally grown. You just have to decide whether the potential benefits from organics are worth the extra money you put down at the cash register.

Organic = Healthier. Not So Fast.

People assume that simply because a food is labeled organic, it's healthier than the conventional alternative. *Wrong!* Organic, as discussed earlier in this chapter, only describes the ingredients and method of production of the food. The labeling says nothing about the healthiness of the food. There are many reasons organics are now a $16 billion industry and one of them is that consumers mistakenly believe that just because they're buying an organic product, they are buying the healthiest item on the shelves. Many, in fact, believe that consuming a diet higher in organic products means that their chance of weight-loss success is greater. Unfortunately, deceptive marketing practices and lack of consumer knowledge has led to many of these misperceptions.

The USDA has purposely remained on the sidelines when it comes to the health claims that are made regarding organic food. They've made it very clear that just because they are the organization responsible for certifying organic food, they by no means make or support any claims that suggest these products are safer, more nutritious, or health-promoting. Even the Organic Farming Research Foundation, which has a stated mission "to foster the improvement and widespread adoption of organic farming systems," agrees that the definitive study looking at whether organics are healthier has yet to be done.

What has been one of the major issues, however, is the amount of pesticide residue that's sitting on or within our food products. This has been most relevant when considering the quality of our fruits and vegetables. Given the devastation that bacteria and other bugs can wreak on crops, farmers have increasingly used pesticides to ward off disease and save their crops. While these chemical bug killers can do an excellent job of protecting crops, the question is what are these pesticides doing to us if we eat them as part of our food.

The active ingredients in pesticides have been shown to cause a series of potential health problems in humans, including nervous system disorders, skin and eye irritation, cancer, hormonal imbalances, and disruption of the endocrine system (responsible for production and release of hormones that influence the functioning of specific organs). But what is not known is whether the amount of pesticides that remain in and on foods sold in supermarkets is enough to cause us biological harm.

The Environmental Protection Agency (EPA) determines what pesticides are acceptable for farming use. Before approving a pesticide, the EPA sets limits on how the pesticide may be used, how often it may be used, and what protective clothing or equipment must be used, and so on. There's an understanding that while fruits and vegetables may be washed before they leave the farm, there is still going to be some pesticide that clings to the outer skin of the food or actually gets into the food itself. This is what is called "pesticide residue." The EPA sets a "tolerance" or maximum residue limit. If residue levels are found to be above the tolerance level, the food item is subject to seizure by the government. When setting the tolerance level, the EPA must make a safety finding that the pesticide can be used with "reasonable certainty of no harm." This tolerance applies to food imported into this country as well as food grown on U.S. soil.

Organic foods are grown without pesticides, and shouldn't have pesticide residue on or in them. This is one reason why some claim organic foods to be healthier. However, there is an argument made from the other side that the amount of pesticide residue that's allowed and found on conventionally farmed products is so low that it does not pose any serious health risk. Many experts come down in the middle of this argument. There is no hard scientific data that conclusively demonstrates conventional farming products are dangerous because of pesticide residue. However, if you can afford to purchase foods that have no chance of containing residue, then why not?

The other issue beyond pesticide residue concerns whether organic foods have higher concentrations of healthy nutrients such as vitamins, minerals, and antioxidants. No large, credible, reproducible studies have been conducted that have shown growing foods organically automatically gives them a boost in any of these nutrients. This is why buying organic food on the premise that you are going to live a better quality of life because you're eating a better quality of food is simply not supported by the facts.

What to Buy Organic

Most experts agree that at the end of the day deciding to buy organic is really a personal preference. There are no guidelines from a leading health organization that spell out which types of food products you should buy organic and which it doesn't make a different. One general rule of thumb I like to follow is that if it's a product that you and/or your family consume a lot of, and you have the disposable income to do so, then it might be to your advantage to purchase organic. While it might not give you a tremendous health advantage over conventional foods or add years to your life, in the worst-case scenario it won't do any harm.

If you want to avoid the hormones and antibiotics that are quite commonplace in our meats, poultry, and dairy these days, then going organic is a way to get these chemicals out of your diet.

The other major criterion that people use to determine whether it makes sense to purchase organic or not is looking at pesticide residue levels. The idea is simple. We know that the pesticides used in our foods find their way into our bodies and can have adverse health effects. This can be especially true for very young infants whose immune systems are still immature and developing. Infants (birth to one year) are fed solids starting at 6 months and in some cases earlier. They're fed pureed fruits and veggies, which makes them vulnerable to more than milk pesticide contamination. A nonprofit organization called the Environmental Working Group has published a widely used list of conventional products and their corresponding levels of pesticide residue. The idea is that if you are concerned about pesticides and their potential harmful effects and you're deciding where you should spend your organic dollars, it's probably wise to purchase the organic variations of those products that tend to have higher pesticide residues. Note, however, that industry experts are quick to point out that even the highest pesticide levels found on these conventional products still fall within the USDA-guided safe range.

Below is a chart of some of the products that typically have high pesticide residue, and thus items that might be high on your organic shopping list. Following that list are items that tend to have very low pesticide residue, so buying the organic alternatives of these products might not give you the biggest bang for your buck. Those items that are at higher risk for retaining pesticide residue are often referred to as "the dirty dozen." If you're going to purchase organic produce, these are the items that should be at the top of your list. This is where chemicals tend to hide.

Great Bang for Your Buck

Apples	Peaches
Celery	Pears
Cherries	Potatoes
Grapes	Spinach
Lettuce	Strawberries
Nectarines	Sweet bell peppers

Not So Great Bang for Your Buck

Asparagus	Mangoes
Avocados	Onions
Bananas	Papayas
Broccoli	Pineapple
Cabbage	Sweet corn
Kiwi	Sweet peas

Not everyone can afford to buy or wants to eat organic foods. This decision does not mean that you are jeopardizing your health. The vast majority of us don't eat anything organic and our health has not suf-fered one bit. But if you are someone who usually purchases conven-tional products and you want to still be the absolute safest, there are a few things you can do to alleviate your worries.

1. Try to buy fruits and vegetables that are in season. If you can purchase produce on the same day it was delivered to the market, all the better. In fact, you can even ask the grocer what day different produce arrives so that you have a better sense of what's freshest.

2. Wash all fresh fruits and vegetables thoroughly with warm running water to reduce the amount of dirt, bacteria, and pesticide residue that might still be clinging to the outer skin. Don't be afraid to use a little scrub brush—a dedicated toothbrush can also do the trick—on products in which you eat the outer skin (apples, cucumbers, pears, potatoes, etc.).

3. Read and understand your labels carefully. Organic products do not mean that the food contains fewer calories, fat, sugar, or salt. Remember the definitions and guidelines that come with organic certification.

4. Peel that skin. If you are really concerned about the pesticide residue that might still be on the produce, peel the fruits and vegetables and trim outer leaves of leafy vegetables as well as wash thoroughly. Be mindful that many nutrients and fiber are found in the outer skin; by peeling it, you might incidentally be reducing the amount of healthy nu-trients you consume. And remember, pesticides as well as hormones and antibiotics reside in fat. If you're eating poultry and/or fish, think about removing the fat from the meat and skin.

You are now armed with enough information to be more knowledge-able in your decision to purchase organic foods or those that have been conventionally farmed. Be a wise consumer and make a decision based on the facts, not the hype machine or rumor mill.

EAT Plan

◆ Choose organic when it makes sense. Just because organic is stamped on the label doesn't mean that product is any healthier than the nonorganic selection. There are certain types of food that make sense to buy organic when you can. Remember the "dirty dozen" when you're shopping, and you'll get more bang for your buck when you go organic.

◆ Many people complain that organic fruits and vegetables spoil much faster than conventional produce. There might be some truth to this given all of the antibiotics and other chemicals that are added to lengthen the shelf life of food. But one way to ensure that you're getting the freshest selections is to check with the produce manager of your store and find out when the food items that you want to purchase are delivered. You can then start buying your organic items on that day.

◆ If you're trying to stretch your dollar, consider buying store-brand organic foods. Just like designer jeans and other designer accessories, the name brands tend to be more expensive. And check the advertisers' coupon/specials. Many of us ignore these promotions, but they really can save you a lot of money, especially when it comes to the organics.

10

The Perfect Snack

- ✦ Snacker's Disasters
- ✦ The Power Snacks
- ✦ Snack Your Way to Weight Loss
- ✦ Snacks for 150 Calories or Less
- ✦ The Mighty Protein Snacks

I'm sick and tired of snacks getting a bad rap. I love snacks. They're awesome. We all should enjoy their gifts. So I tried to figure out why snacks seem to be the enemy in so many people's minds, and I think I found a couple of answers. First, a lot of people don't understand what a snack is and what purpose it's supposed to serve. Second, too many people are out of control and ruin snacking's reputation by taking a good thing way too far.

A snack is defined by most dictionaries as "a small quantity of food;

a light meal or refreshment taken between regular meals." I like to think of a snack as a bridge between meals, a way to satisfy the body's growing hunger until it's time to sit down and eat a larger meal. Snacks are not meant to replace meals. Snacks are not meant to be free-for-alls when you consume close to or as many calories as you would at a regular meal. A snack is meant to be small and finite.

Unfortunately, just as with restaurant food and package size, we have distorted the portion size and frequency of our snacks. Too many of us sit down for a snack and easily consume 600 to 800 calories, the same amount or even more than what we should be typically consuming for an *entire* meal. Just do the numbers. A couple of snacks at that rate means that you could be consuming half of your day's calorie count before you've eaten even one meal!

What should you be looking for in a snack? The first place to start is calories. Snacks should be from 150 to 200 calories. This is enough calories for your body to know that it's been fed something, but not so many calories that your body thinks it's had a complete meal. The snack shouldn't fill you up, but just take the edge off the hunger that's growing within. You want to beat back the distracting growls in your stomach not to the point that they disappear, but so that they become nothing more than a whimper.

The frequency of your snacks is also critical. The average person can do just fine on three snacks a day. If your snacks are extremely light (100 calories or less), then you can have even more. You should be strategic not just with the content of your snacks, but with the timing of your snacks. Use them as a way to stretch your hunger tolerance until you have the opportunity to sit down and eat a real meal. Smart eating says eating four small- to moderate-sized meals is the best way to distribute your calories throughout the day and prevent hormonal spikes that can occur in response to ingesting a big meal. Your snacking should complement these meals so that there's no point throughout the day where you are overwhelmed with hunger.

Planning is key. Just as it's important to plan your meals, it's also important to plan your snacks. Taking a few minutes to think about what you will be eating and stocking up on those items can be critical, especially if you're going to find yourself in an environment where your choices are limited. The workplace is a great example. Many vending machines are loaded with nothing but bad choices: sugary foods full of empty calories. But often these machines are our only source of snacks when we don't have the time to go find a store with a bigger, healthier selection. So the only options left are not eating a snack at all or choosing something from the vending machine. Both options are less than optimal. It's so much easier to bring snacks with you. Either prepare and bag them at home or stop and purchase them on your way to work. Knowing what you'll be eating in advance gives you peace of mind that you won't be desperately running from vending machine to vending machine trying to figure out the best choices out of the worst options or grabbing the doughnuts sitting next to the coffeemaker.

The perfect snack does three important things: (1) it settles some of the hunger impulse that's causing your stomach to growl and causing you to think about food above other tasks you might be trying to perform; (2) it gives you a small dose of whatever the taste or sensation is that you're craving; (3) it gives you a little shot of energy that doesn't have you doing cartwheels, but gives you a pick-me-up you might need until you have a chance to sit down to a full meal.

When choosing a snack there are also things you should avoid. Here is your cheat sheet:

1. **Avoid trans fats.** Trans fats have gotten a lot of negative publicity lately and for good reason. Trans fats, also called hydrogenated oils or partially

hydrogenated oils, raise the bad cholesterol (LDL) and lower the good cholesterol (HDL). They are often found in snacks such as crackers, cakes, pies, cookies, and frozen fried microwave snacks, among others. Look for the terms "trans fat," "hydrogenated oil," or "partially hydrogenated oil" in the ingredients. If you see any of these terms, leave that product on the shelf. Sometimes manufacturers make it easier for you by labeling their products "0 trans fats," or "no trans fats."

2. **Beware of energy bars.** There are hundreds of "energy" or "power" bars that are being heavily marketed as a convenient, nutritious way to boost your energy and get a quick dose of healthy calories. But remember that all bars are not created equal. Yes, the portability of these bars make them universally convenient, but take a quick look at the calories they contain as well as some of the other ingredients, such as fat and sugar. You should try for a bar that has 3 to 5 grams of fiber, 5 to 10 grams of protein, lower amounts of fat (no saturated fat), less than 15 grams of sugar, and no more than 200 calories. You might not be able to meet all of these requirements with one bar, but try to get as close as you can.

3. **Avoid reflex snacking.** Don't snack simply because you think it's time to snack or because you see that snack food is available. Snacks are meant to be eaten strategically—you eat them when you need them and they help you immediately satisfy hunger impulses. If you don't need the extra calories, why consume them? Mindless eating occurs when people eat just to eat even when they're not hungry and often when they're doing something else, such as watching a movie or working at the computer. Make your snacks count, but don't abuse them.

4. **Avoid high-fat snacks.** The first reason is obvious. Higher-fat snacks tend to be higher in calories and lower in more healthful nutrients. Another reason to avoid them is the natural tendency we have to over-

consume fatty foods. We seem to have a more difficult time cutting ourselves off when it comes to fatty snacks and find ourselves eating multiple servings instead of one.

Salty Snacks

These are some of the most highly desired snacks. Yet they can also be of the most concern, because too much salt can have adverse consequences, such as increasing water retention and elevating blood pressure. So the trick is to satisfy that salt craving without consuming too much salt or too many calories. Try these salty snacks, which are all under 150 calories.

8 Reduced-Fat Triscuit crackers

27 Snyder's of Hanover Mini Pretzels

$\frac{1}{4}$ cup (1 ounce) dry-roasted pumpkin seeds in shell

$\frac{3}{4}$ cup edamame

Olives (black, 10–15) (green, 1 cup)

Buffalo mozzarella (1 ounce), cherry or grape tomatoes ($\frac{1}{2}$ cup)

Prosciutto (30 grams), dried figs (3)

Baked potato chips (100-calorie bag)

7 Saltine crackers

Popcorn, air popped (3 cups, lightly salted)

Melba toast (4 slices)

Sweet Snacks

1 Balance Bar (100 calories)

Original Apple Nature Valley Fruit Crisps (1 package)

continued

1 cup of unsweetened apple sauce with a sprinkle of cinnamon

1 small brownie (2" by 1")

3 small chocolate chip cookies

Graham crackers (2 squares and 2 teaspoons of low-sugar jelly)

Sugar-free chocolate pudding ($1/2$ cup) with 1 tablespoon of whipped topping

$1/2$ cup of fat-free ice cream

Low-fat yogurt (8 ounces)

1 cup orange juice (frozen) and eat with a spoon

Graham cracker (1) with marshmallow on top (microwave until gooey) and chocolate syrup (1 teaspoon)

Frozen seedless grapes (15)

Fresh cherries (20)

1 medium orange (sliced)

1 Dole fruit bar

2 Good Humor Fat Free Fudgsicle

2 sugar-free Popsicles

Apricots, dried (8 halves)

Strawberries (5 sliced) with 1 tablespoon of whipped cream

Frozen yogurt ($1/2$ cup)

Sliced bananas and fresh raspberries (1 cup)

Pineapple-Raspberry Yogurt Parfait (8 ounces fat-free yogurt, $1/2$ cup pineapple chunks, $1/2$ cup of raspberries)

Crunchy Snacks

Hummus ($1/4$ cup) and small bag of baby carrots

Celery (3 stalks) and 1 tablespoon of peanut butter

10 cashews

10 to 14 almonds

Raw veggies (1 cup of red bell peppers, celery, 1 cup carrot sticks) and
  fat-free salad dressing ($\frac{1}{4}$ cup)

Apple ($\frac{1}{2}$ cut into slices) and peanut butter (2 teaspoons)

Dill pickles

Whole wheat pita bread, toasted and sliced into triangles, and 2
  tablespoons of low-fat hummus

Low-fat Kettle Crisps

Nabisco Ginger Snap Cookies (4)

Cucumber slices (15) with 1 tablespoon of low-fat or fat-free dressing

Wheat Thin crackers (4) and 1 ounce of cheese

4 mini rice cakes with 2 tablespoons of low-fat cottage cheese

5 ounces tossed salad (lettuce, tomato, cucumber, carrot slices),
  $\frac{1}{4}$ cup fat-free dressing

Chocolate

15 chocolate-covered raisins

5 strawberries (medium) dipped into 1 ounce melted dark chocolate
  chips

Whole-grain chocolate chip cookies

Low-fat Fudgsicle

Fat-free chocolate yogurt

1 cup of Chocolate Cheerios

Quaker chocolate rice cakes

Jell-O sugar-free chocolate pudding cup

Curves chocolate peanut bar

Health Valley chocolate chip granola bar

Protein Snacks

Snacking can be an optimal time to increase your protein intake. There are many foods that pack a powerful protein punch without jumping out of the calorie range we're trying to maintain. Protein is a key snack ingredient because it has fewer calories than some of the fattier snacks and it requires more energy for the body to digest it, which means it also causes the body to burn calories. Try some of these protein snacks when your stomach starts to growl.

Tuna. Make sure you get tuna in water. A small can typically contains less than 120 calories and is fat free. Each can delivers as much as 25 grams of protein. It's fine to mix the tuna with condiments like mayonnaise, but keep them to a minimum. These are where you start stacking up on hidden calories.

Protein Bars. The first thing you need to know is that not all protein bars are created equal. There are hundreds of brands and types on the market, but you need to be a smart consumer when deciding which is best for you. You want to make sure that your protein bar is high in protein (of course) and low in carbohydrates and fats. When selecting your protein bar snack, aim for those numbers previously listed for energy bars (see page 174).

Turkey Roll-Ups. These are easy to make and full of protein. Take a piece of turkey and cut it into thin strips. Then take pieces of low-fat cheese and lay them on top of the turkey strips. Roll up the turkey so that the cheese is in the middle. This convenient snack provides plenty of protein and is low in calories.

Cottage Cheese. This is an excellent source of protein and easy to eat as a snack. There are 16 grams in half a cup and only 90 calories. Put it on rice cakes or fruit and you have a healthy protein snack with a low-calorie cost.

Roast Beef Sandwich. Three and a half ounces of roast beef delivers approximately 28 grams of protein. Add it to a slice of bread, low-fat mayonnaise, and half a slice of low-fat cheese and you'll have plenty of protein for under 200 calories.

Roasted Chickpeas. An excellent source of protein without consuming too many calories. Low in fat and high in fiber, half a cup of chickpeas will fill you up and deliver such nutrients as iron and folate. Sprinkle some salt on them as they roast and satisfy the craving you might have for something salty.

Whatever you decide to eat as a snack, try to approach snacking with the right frame of mind. Rather than looking at snacks as an opportunity to cheat in a small way that you can get away with, think about snacks as opportunities. You have the chance to get in more fruits and vegetables and fill up on foods that will not only beat back the hunger, but will deliver some health benefits. Sometimes you simply have a craving for something that's completely unhealthy, perhaps your favorite junk food that you know has little if any nutritional value at all. No one's perfect, nor is anyone expected to be perfect. Go ahead and have a little bit of what you're craving, but remember it's all about moderation. A snack, even if it's not the healthiest, is still a snack. You don't want to go so far off the deep end that you end up adding another meal's worth of calories to your day with little to show for it. Snacks are *awesome*!

EAT Plan

◆ Plan on eating three snacks per day. Two of your snacks should be 150 calories or less and at least one of these snacks needs to be crunchy. Your third snack can be less healthy (potato chips, brownie, ice cream, etc.), but it must still be less than 200 calories.

◆ The timing of these snacks is also important. Snacks are best eaten with a strategy. Do not eat your snacks consecutively or all at once as this defeats the purpose of the snack. Remember, a snack is a bridge between meals. If you want to eat a snack, try to do so at least an hour after a meal or an hour before a meal.

◆ Make sure you drink a cup (8 ounces) or more of water (or another beverage that is low in calories or contains no calories at all) with your snack. Your next meal should come an hour or more after consuming your snack. Your snacking would look something like this:

8:00 AM	10:00 AM	12:00 PM	3:00 PM	4:30 PM	7:00 PM
	8:30 PM				
Meal 1	Snack 1	Meal 2	Meal 3	Snack 2	Meal 3
	Snack 3				

Strategic Eating 11

> ✦ Shed the Pounds
>
> ✦ Build Muscle
>
> ✦ Fight Diabetes
>
> ✦ Surviving the Holidays
>
> ✦ Suppress Your Appetite
>
> ✦ Downsize for Better Eating

*A*ll of us must eat for the basic nourishment of our bodies so that we can live and carry out our daily activities. But there are times we eat with other purposes, whether it's losing weight, training for a marathon, trying to gain muscle, or fighting disease. What we eat and how we eat it can make a big difference in the quality and length of our life. This chapter is designed to help you achieve your goals through strategic eating. Rather than having to follow a difficult, rigid plan, the following sections will guide you through the earlier information in the book and show how to best use it to achieve your goals.

Weight Loss

Your focus chapters are 1, 2, 3, 4, 7, 8, and 10. The **EAT Plan** at the end of these chapters, if followed, will produce considerable weight loss in a relatively short period of time. The eleven changes in the following box can help you achieve the results you desire. But remember that adding a regimen of physical activity/exercise will magnify your weight loss. Attempt to get in 30 to 45 minutes of moderate intensity physical activity 3 to 5 days a week. Start off slowly if you're unaccustomed to exercise, then build your way up until you can go 45 minutes five days a week. Always check with your doctor first, of course, before beginning any exercise program.

Strategic Eating for Weight Loss

✦ Consume at least 5 servings of fruits and vegetables each day. If you can get more in by all means do so. Start and end your day with a piece of fruit. Try to alternate your fruits between days. Berries are your best friends. Full of antioxidants and other nutrients, berries can fill you up on fewer calories and provide a natural sweetness. Eat them in yogurt and blend them in smoothies. Half of your plate at every meal should be fruits and veggies. Refer to chapter 1 for an overview of healthy eating.

✦ Choose fruits that are low on the glycemic index. At least half of your fruits for the day should come from this list: cherries (raw sour), grapefruit, apricots (dried), apples, pears, plums, peaches, kiwi, oranges, grapes. Refer to chapter 1 for more information on the glycemic index scale.

◆ Go brown! Reduce or eliminate white bread, white pasta, white potatoes (determined by the color of the pulp, not the skin), and white rice. Replace these with the browns—100% whole-grain bread, whole wheat pasta, yams or sweet potatoes, brown rice. Refer to chapter 3.

◆ Dairy can provide great health benefits, but be mindful of the calorie load. Switch your dairy from regular to fat-free, 1% fat, or reduced-fat products. Just making this switch can save you a few hundred calories each day. Refer to chapter 5 for the chart on milk and dairy products.

◆ Whenever possible, load up on whole grains. You should consume at least 3 servings (48 grams) each day. Refer to chapter 3 to find out which foods contain the best whole grains.

◆ Fill up on fiber. You will eat less and feel full longer. Aim for 25 to 30 grams of fiber each day. Refer to chapter 4 to find those foods that are the most fiber-rich.

◆ Try eating most of your meals on a salad-sized plate. Don't pile the food more than half an inch high. Refer to chapter 7 for a visual presentation of what a serving size looks like.

◆ Water will fill you up with no calories and will help flush your kidneys. Drink at least 6 cups of water each day. At least half of what you drink each day should be water. Start and end the day with a cup of water. Have at least one cup of water at each meal. Refer to chapter 8 for the benefits of drinking water.

◆ Try to consume no more than 3 snacks each day and make sure these snacks are no more than 150 to 200 calories. Eat them between meals and make sure each snack for the day is different. One day might be popcorn, grapes, and baby carrots. Another day might be

continued

3 chocolate chip cookies, apple slices, and rice cakes with cottage cheese. Refer to chapter 10 to learn about proper snacks.

✦ Divide your meals into 4 small- to moderate-sized meals each day. Space them approximately 3 hours apart and bridge them with snacks. Refer to chapters 7 and 10.

✦ If you're trying to lose weight and thus counting calories—and I'm not saying you have to—try keeping your calories within a certain range. This is a gross generalization, but for women attempt 1,100 to 1,400 calories; for men 1,300 to 1,600 calories. Once again, these are only ranges and your unique variables (height, weight, weight-loss goal, amount of lean muscle, physical activity, etc.) will determine where you land. But as a general rule, eat enough calories so that you're not hungry, but not too many to the point of feeling stuffed. Refer to chapter 7.

Muscle Building

You don't have to be a body builder to want to increase your lean muscle mass. Muscle is important for more reasons than just looking good in front of a mirror or on the beach. Muscles can increase your metabolism, thus increase your calorie burn. They can also make you more resilient when you suffer an illness and need to recover. Physical activity is critical to increasing your muscle mass. Specifically, resistance training is the best exercise to get your muscles pumping. You might try resistance bands, but also try free weights, which give you your biggest muscle bang for your buck. Women benefit from lifting free weights just as much as men do. The old belief that lifting weights was a man's exercise is simply wrong and outdated. Safe and effective weight lifting can provide the fastest and most efficient way to increase your muscle. You should be focusing on chapters 2, 4, 5, 7, and 10.

Strategic Eating for Muscle Building

◆ Carbs are important when building muscle mass. Bad carbs can work against your efforts, so it's critical to focus on the good carbs listed in chapter 2. Make sure 75 percent of your carbs come from the good list.

◆ Fiber is important in helping to keep your colon clean as well as answering your increased hunger due to the development of hungry muscle. Strive for at least 30 grams of fiber each day. Chapter 4 will give you those fiber-rich foods.

◆ Protein is critical for you. Protein is the building block of muscle. It's critical that you have a healthy and plentiful supply of protein. Attempt to consume 65 to 80 grams of protein each day. Chapter 5 will give you the best sources of protein. Remember to load up on the "healthy" protein, such as chicken and fish. These types of protein sources will give you the protein you need without loading you up on calories that can lead to increasing your fat mass.

◆ Just like those who are trying to lose weight, portion sizes matter for you also. If you're trying to build muscle, you will need to consume more calories than the person trying to lose weight, which means your portion sizes should be slightly larger. You want to gain muscle mass, which means also increasing your calories. Remember, there are 3,500 calories per pound, so if you are trying to gain a pound of muscle, that's going to take some work. In general, you should try consuming at least 3,000 healthy, proteinaceous calories each day. This is taking into account that you will be exercising and thus burning off some of these calories.

◆ Snack on things that are high in protein, low in fat, and energy dense. Don't waste your snack calories on things like cookies and chips. Instead, consider protein bars, granola, oatmeal, peanut butter, and leafy green veggies. You should consume 4 snacks per day as well as 4 meals per day.

Preventing and Fighting Diabetes

More than 26 million Americans suffer from type 2 diabetes, an illness that is often associated with obesity as well as poor eating and exercise habits. There are an estimated 50 to 60 million pre-diabetics in the United States—these are people who aren't yet diabetic but right on the fence. The bad news about type 2 diabetes is that the number of afflicted continues to rise, and now even our children and adolescents are developing a disease that was once only seen in adults. The bodily harm this illness causes is widespread and debilitating. But that leads to the good news. Diabetes in many cases is preventable and manageable, and one does not have to be on medications to control it. Changes in physical activity levels and eating behaviors can go a long way in helping diabetics improve their blood sugar levels.

No two diabetics are the same. It can be a largely idiosyncratic illness, which is why each diabetic must be familiar with his or her own disease. A certain food might cause a glucose spike in one person and not another. Because of this, it's impossible to prescribe a highly specified diabetic diet. We now know after much research that regular physical activity is quite beneficial for diabetics. I have witnessed this firsthand in patients and members of my own family. We also know that there are some basic nutritional guidelines that can make a difference in most diabetics. Your focus should be chapters 1, 2, 3, 4, 7, 8, and 10.

Strategic Eating for Preventing and Fighting Diabetes

◆ Experiment with a variety of fruits and vegetables and figure out which ones cause a fast spike in your blood glucose levels and which ones don't. Keep a list of the "good" vs. "bad" fruits and veggies as they pertain to your diabetes.

◆ Avoid as many white, starchy foods as possible. Whole grains are your best friends. From cereals to breads to pasta, enjoy the taste and healthy advantages of whole grains and leave behind the high glycemic index carbs that can wreak havoc on your blood glucose levels.

◆ Fiber can be very beneficial to diabetics as it can reduce the level of glucose in the blood. Consume at least 35 grams of fiber each day. Make sure the fiber-rich foods you choose are those that work well with your diabetic eating plan.

◆ Portion control is critical for diabetics. Keeping the calorie loads in your meals evenly balanced is important to prevent erratic insulin spikes. Don't eat heavy meals; instead, divide your calories between 4 or 5 meals throughout the day. Despite the temptation, don't skip meals as this can cause dangerous fluctuations in your sugar levels.

◆ Sugary liquids are a no no, and even juices might be a problem for you as they can lead to a quick rise in blood glucose levels. Try to drink 75 percent of your fluids in the form of water and flavor it with chunks of fresh fruit if desired. Limit your alcohol consumption to no more than one drink per day. Alcohol can be extremely harmful for diabetics.

◆ Your choice of snacks is critical as hidden calories and added sugars can cause serious problems with your ability to properly regulate blood glucose levels. Make sure that half of your snacks have fiber or whole grains. Vegetables snacks are excellent for diabetics, so make sure that at least two of your day's snacks involve fresh veggies.

continued

✦ Make sure that most of the fats you consume are unsaturated. Also, avoid trans fats at all costs. Diabetes can make you more susceptible to blood vessel and heart disease. You don't want to complicate the situation by eating bad fats that will only increase your risk for clogged arteries.

Surviving the Holidays

Holidays are a wonderful time to share quality time with family and other loved ones. It's also a wonderful opportunity to eat great-tasting foods and lots of them. Contrary to what most experts will tell you, I believe that people should have fun eating during holidays and other social occasions. It's a great time to eat those dishes you rarely get a chance to eat or you've been refraining from eating because it's full of calories and not in accordance with your weight-loss plan.

Well, I believe you should go for it. Cakes, macaroni and cheese, fried foods, have all of it. But there's a way to eat these faves without breaking the scale. Here are some tips to make it through the holiday enjoying your food, but not packing on those extra pounds.

Strategic Eating for Surviving the Holidays

✦ A holiday is a day, *not* 3 days or a week. Sure, you might be in the fes-tive spirit for more than a day, and that's completely fine. But that prolonged festive spirit should not lead to prolonged holiday eating. Eat all of those foods on the actual day, but don't continue that type and volume of eating over the next 3 or 4 days. This is where people lose control and start packing on extra pounds.

✦ Build a reserve. If you know that you're going to splurge during a holiday, then prepare for it. Three weeks before the holiday be especially vigilant when it comes to eating well and exercising. If you lose a couple of pounds before the holiday, then at worst you'll be even after the holidays. Building a cushion before the holidays allows you to be less restricted during your time of celebration.

◆ Alternate meals. If you know that you're going to be enjoying foods that aren't exactly the healthiest, then reach a compromise. Alternate healthy meals with those that are not so healthy. This will still allow you to enjoy your favorite foods without overindulging.

◆ Advance eating. If you know that you're going to a holiday party where high-calorie food and drinks are going to be served, there's still a way to participate without doing harm. Eat a small amount of food an hour before going to the party. By the time you get there, you'll still be hungry enough to want to enjoy some of the offerings, but you won't be so hungry that you'll gorge on all of those fattening calories.

◆ Split your dinner. If you know that there will be lots of foods that you want to eat for dinner, rather than eat one large meal, divide it into two. Eat a lighter plate earlier than your typical dinnertime, then eat another serving a couple of hours later. This will help keep your blood sugar and hormone levels even.

Suppress Your Appetite

One strategy in trying to prevent overeating is to naturally suppress your appetite. You've certainly heard commercials on the radio or TV touting special "appetite suppressant" pills that supposedly decrease your hunger. Unfortunately, many of these products are nothing more than gimmicks that have not been scientifically tested or contain unidentified ingredients whose short- and long-term health effects are unknown.

There are, however, natural ways to suppress your appetite and the most well documented come in the form of the types of food you eat. In general, foods that combine protein, fiber, and/or other complex carbo-hydrates tend to trick your body into believing that it no longer is as hungry as it was before you started eating. A great example is a slice of whole-grain bread spread with peanut butter. Another combination is apple and peanut butter. Take slices of apples and dip them in peanut butter. The idea is simple. When we respond to our hunger by eating healthier and more nutritiously valuable food, then we diminish our cravings for junk food, which gives us the shortest hunger relief for the maximum number of calories.

Pine Nuts. These nuts contain the highest amount of protein of any other seed. When we consume protein-rich foods, messages are sent to our hormonal system that effectively tell the brain that we're full. These nuts also contain what's believed to be a potent appetite suppressant ingredient: pinolenic acid. This naturally occurring polyunsaturated fat works by stimulating two powerful hunger-suppressing hormones—cholecystokinin (CCK) and glucagon-like peptide-1 (GLP-1). Here's the skinny: CCK is released by the first portion of our intestines once a partially digested meal rich in fats or protein leaves the stomach. CCK then acts to slow down the amount of time our stomach takes to empty and thus promotes a feeling of fullness, which then suppresses further food intake. GLP-1 delivers its effect in a similar manner. It, too, is pro-duced in the small intestine, but in response to a meal that contains fat and carbohydrates. It works by slowing down the absorption of food in the gut, which promotes feelings of fullness and satiety. The end result is that it limits our desire to continue eating. One study presented at a meeting of the American Chemical Society showed that participants who consumed higher amounts of pinolenic acid reduced their food intake by an impressive 36 percent.[1]

Apples. You can never tire of touting the wonders of apples. Be-yond its dentist-resistant properties, it is a perfect snack. An apple is a great source of fiber, which is a natural appetite-suppressant. High-fiber foods generally require more chewing time, so eating them gives your body extra time to register that you're no longer hungry. With feelings of hunger diminished, you're less likely to overeat. (That's another reason why apples are such an excellent snack.) They're low in calories (100 or less typically) and low in fat. They're also very portable, easy to maintain, and inexpensive.

Oatmeal. This old standby is a great example of what an appetite-suppressing snack should contain. Comprised of carbohydrate and fiber (among other things) it has that special combination that makes you feel full. The other advantage of oatmeal is that it has a low glycemic index (a measure of how quickly foods are converted to sugar once digested), which means sugar enters your bloodstream slower, keeping you full for a longer time. Oatmeal has long been touted for its cholesterol-lowering effects, up to 23 percent in some studies. To get all of the benefits of oatmeal there is one catch, however: it's better to eat the real stuff, not the instant. Just 1 cup can pack a mighty nutritional punch.

Flaxseeds. While flaxseed sounds like something new on the nutritional scene, it's anything but. Cultivated in Babylon as early as 3000 BC, it's considered one of the most powerful plant foods on the planet. Among many of its purported health benefits, there is some evidence that it can help reduce the risk of cancer, diabetes, heart disease, and stroke. Flaxseed owes its healthy reputation to three major ingredients: (1) fiber—it contains both the soluble and insoluble types; (2) omega-3 essential fatty acids—also known as the "good" fats that have been shown in many studies to have benefits on reducing the risk for heart disease; and (3) lignans—chemical compounds that have both plant estrogen and antioxidant qualities. Flaxseed can contain up to 800 times more lignans than other plant foods. You can add flaxseed to other foods such as oatmeal, smoothies, soup, or yogurt. You can also use ground flaxseed as part of the flour that's called for in recipes for breads, muffins, waffles, and pancakes. Flaxseed can be purchased whole or ground (milled). To receive the more complete benefit of flaxseed, opt for the ground form because your body is better able to digest it. You can also grind it at home in a clean electric coffee grinder.

Drinks. As boring as it might sound, water can be an excellent appetite suppressant. Just as little as 8 ounces can settle your stomach during the early stages of hunger. Also consider blended drinks such as protein shakes, soy-based drinks, and fat-free milk shakes. Blending protein powder or real fruit into a shake can be appetizing and filling at the same time. Make sure, however, that you watch your calorie count along the way. If you're drinking your snack instead of eating it, stay mindful of how many calories you're consuming.

Downsizing for a Bigger Life

In a perfect world we could sit down to the table and tell our stomach and brain to only consume a certain amount of food that falls neatly into a healthy caloric range. Well, we don't live in a perfect world, so we have to strategize ways to curb our appetites and resist going back to the fridge or stove for seconds. Remembering the principle that the stomach and brain communicate by the stretch concept can help you develop ways to reduce the volume of what you eat. When we're hungry the brain sends a signal out instructing us to find food and eat, so we pick up food and start eating. The more food we eat, the more our stomach is stretched. When our stomach is stretched to a certain point, a signal is sent from the stomach to the brain's satiety center telling it that we're satisfied and there's no need to continue eating. There are also hormones that are released or prevented from being released to signal an impulse to stop eating. (Unfortunately, many of us override this signal, and despite the fact that we're full, continue to eat in excess.)

So the trick is to satisfy our hunger, but doing so on fewer calories. One way that has been helpful to those I've worked with is to get them to choose those foods and beverages that are lower in calories that can stretch the stomach and send the "I'm full" signal to the brain. One of the easiest and least expensive ways to do this is using good old-fashioned water. You can reduce the amount of food you need to fill up your stomach by drinking a cup of water before your meal, a cup during your meal, and a cup before dessert. Try squeezing a fresh lemon in the water to give it some flavor without adding any calories.

Another useful strategy that can help you control the portions you consume of those high-calorie foods is to eat most of your vegetables and other low-calorie foods first. Save those high-calorie items like French fries, heavy creams, and rich sauces for the end of the meal when you're more likely to be full and less likely to eat all of them.

Another simple way to downsize is to take your time. One of the problems with our eating habits—or overeating habits—is that we always seem to be in a rush. Either we're eating in the car on our way to work, running out the door, or between appointments. Too many of us have gotten away from sitting down and enjoying our food in good company. This is problematic, because the faster you eat the more you eat. Rapid consumption doesn't give your stomach and brain time to register that you are full and to send the stop-eating signals before you overindulge. It might take on average 20 to 30 minutes after consuming the majority of your meal for your body to start feeling full and registering this satiety in your brain. So after you finish what's on your plate, before reaching for a second helping, take a few minutes and drink something. This will allow your stomach to register its satisfaction with the amount of food you've consumed.

It's also important to know when it's time to remove yourself from a tempting food environment. While it's all right to take your time eating meals, it can be counterproductive if you spend too much time around food after you're finished eating. I've seen this with my own family after a meal. Some of my relatives will stay in the kitchen finishing their conversation. And after they've already put their dishes in the sink, they'll drift to the pots or serving platters and start picking at more food, not because they're hungry, but because it's there and they can see and smell it and it's become a reflex for them to reach out and nibble. It's not that you have to end the conversation you're enjoying, but you can finish your conversation or drinks in another room away from the leftovers, which have an insidious way of beckoning you to come back and get more.

This nibbling while conversing leads to another important issue: "mindless eating." One of our biggest eating behavior mistakes is eating while trying to do other things. Whether it's sitting in your living room watching a movie, working at your computer, or talking on the phone, eating while carrying out other tasks can often lead to overconsumption, because you're typically giving little consideration to how much food you're putting in your mouth. You start off with just a handful of chips and the next thing you know you've consumed the entire bag—all 440 calories! When you're eating, focus on the food and your companions, but avoid as much as possible eating while distracted or when in engaged in other activities.

Afterword

Volumes have been and will be written on healthy eating and the positive impact that good nutrition can play in our lives. In *EAT*, I hope I have given you simple, but critical information that will help you form a strategy to enjoy good food while improving the quality of your life. Unfortunately, too many people mistakenly believe that starving themselves or eliminating entire food groups is the way to eat better, lose weight, and improve their health. *Not so.*

Eating is one of life's greatest experiences, a daily opportunity to explore, discover, indulge, and share. Too often we have little regard or concern or understanding of what we put into our amazing bodies. While our physical package is the greatest machine that's ever been built, it must be cared for and maintained properly to continue to operate at peak performance.

It's often difficult to make sense of the conflicting messages and marketing hype about food that bombard us on a daily basis. I hope that *EAT* has both inspired and informed you, and has made you curious and confident about the fuel that you pump into your body. There is no universal set of nutritional rules that applies to everyone. One of the beauties of life is that we are unique individuals. The combination of our taste preferences and how our bodies process and metabolize certain foods are particular to us. Despite this individuality, however, all of us need to make smart choices. You are now armed with the knowledge to not only master these choices, but also to not be afraid of them.

I devised the **EAT Plan** so that it is not rigid or intimidating, but rather completely accessible and easy to integrate into anyone's life. I wanted to take the guesswork out of the equation for you and provide a blueprint for good eating, a blueprint that you can alter with your own details and specifications as you go along experimenting and learning— and eating! Remember, a large part of nutritional success lies in your willingness to have an open mind, to try new things, and to exhibit a little discipline. You can eat and drink *almost* anything you desire, but moderation is essential. No one eats or lives perfectly and anyone who expects to will be disappointed. But you *can* make changes to what you eat that will *never* make you feel like you're on a diet but will immediately make you feel stronger, more alert, lighter, and more capable. The **EAT Plan** can make a big difference in your life because it doesn't call for perfection. *EAT* is about eating the best that you can and enjoying the benefits—and the taste!—of good food. So, go to your next meal as a critical thinker and discriminating food detective. But most of all, go ahead and EAT!

Notes and Sources

CHAPTER 1: FOLLOW THE RAINBOW

1. Fruits and vegetable consumption among adults—United States, 2005, *Morbidity and Mortality Weekly Reports,* March 16, 2007; 56 (10): 213–17.
2. From the National Academy of Sciences, Institute of Medicine, Food, and Nutrition Board.

CHAPTER 3: THE WHOLE TRUTH ABOUT WHOLE GRAINS

1. Larson et al. Whole-grain intake correlates among adolescents and young adults: Findings from project eat. *Journal of the American Dietetic Association,* 2010; 110 (2): 230.

CHAPTER 4: FEEL FULL FIBER

1. Rimm EB, Ascherio A, Giovannucci E, Spiegelman D, Stampfer MJ, Willett WC. Vegetable, fruit, and cereal fiber intake and risk of coronary heart disease among men. *Journal of the American Medical Association,* 1996; 275: 447–51.
2. Associations between diet and cancer, ischemic heart disease, and all-cause mortality in non-Hispanic white California Seventh-day Adventists. *American Journal of Clinical Nutrition,* September 1999; 70 (3): 532S–538S.
3. Brown L, Rosner B, Willett WW, Sacks FM. Cholesterol-lowering effects of dietary fiber: A mega-analysis. *American Journal of Clinical Nutrition,* January 1999; 69 (1): 30–42.
4. Montonen J, Knekt P, Järvinen R, Aromaa A, Reunanen A. Whole-grain and fiber intake and the incidence of type 2 diabetes. *American Journal of Clinical Nutrition,* March 2003; 77 (3): 622–29.
5. Fuchs CS, Giovannucci EL, Colditz GA, et al. Dietary fiber and the risk of colorectal cancer and adenoma in women. *New England Journal of Medicine,* 1999; 340: 169–76.

CHAPTER 5: PROTEIN BONANZA

1. USDA Nutrient Database for Standard Reference, Release 14. Washington, D.C.: U.S. Department of Agriculture.

2.   Chao A, Thun MJ, Connell CJ, McCullough ML, et al. Meat consumption and risk of colorectal cancer. *Journal of the American Medical Association,* 2005; 293: 172–82.

CHAPTER 6: SPICETOPIA

1.   Silagy C, Neil A. Garlic as a lipid-lowering agent—a meta-analysis. *Journal of the Royal College of Physicians of London.* January–February 1994.
2.   Sobenin IA, et al. Lipid-lowering effects of time-released garlic powder tablets in double-blinded placebo-controlled randomized study. *Journal of the Royal College of Physicians of London.* December 2008.
3.   Murray, MT. *The Healing Powers of Herbs: The Enlightened Person's Guide to the Wonders of Medicinal Plants.*

CHAPTER 7: SIZE MATTERS

1.   Organisation for Economic Cooperation and Development (OECD), Health Statistics, 2004.
2.   See http://www.cdc.gov/needphp/dnpa/nutrition/pdf/portion_size_research.pdf.
3.   McCrory MA, Fuss PJ, Hays NP, Vinken AG, Greenberg AS, Roberts SB. Overeating in America: Association between restaurant food consumption and body fatness in healthy adult men and women. *Obesity Research,* 1999; 7 (6): 564–71.
4.   U.S. Bureau of Labor Statistics, Consumer Expenditure Survey (2004–2005) for four-person households.
5.   Young LR, Nestle M. The contribution of expanding portion sizes to the U.S. obesity epidemic. *American Journal of Public Health,* 2002; 92 (2): 246–49.

CHAPTER 8: YOU ARE WHAT YOU DRINK

1.   Information from the Tea Association of the USA, Inc.
2.   Information from the National Coffee Association.
3.   Sesso HD, Gaziano JM, Buring JE, Hennekens CH. Coffee and tea intake and the risk of myocardial infarction. *American Journal of Epidemiology,* 1999; 149: 162–67.
4.   Davies MJ., Judd JT., et al. Black tea consumption reduces total and LDL cholesterol in widely hypercholesterolemic adults. *Journal of Nutrition,* 2003; 133: 32985–33025.
5.   Davidson TL, Swithers SE. A Pavlovian approach to the problem of obesity. *International Journal of Obesity and Related Metabolic Disorders,* July 2004; 28 (7): 933–35.

CHAPTER 11: STRATEGIC EATING

1.   Causey JL. Korean pine nut fatty acids [pinolenic acid] induce satiety-producing hormone release in overweight human volunteers. Paper presented at American Chemical Society National Meeting & Exposition, March 26–30, 2006, Atlanta, Georgia.

Index

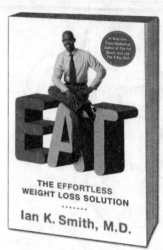
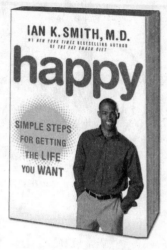
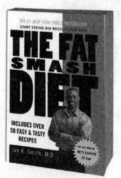
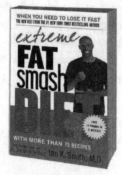
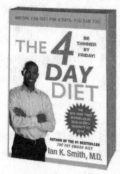

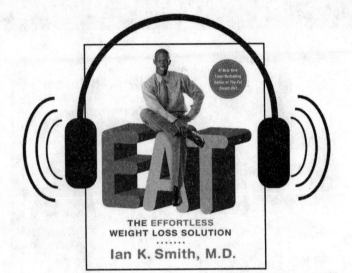